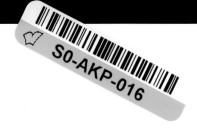

The Yoga Habit

A Manual for Beginners

June Browne

Table of Contents

Introduction

Yoga is a lifestyle and a way of being. It improves your health and sculpts your body, and is so much more than just about getting into a fancy backbend or touching your toes.

Although yoga isn't a religion, it can certainly be a spiritual practice. The very definition of yoga lies in union and connection. It's a way of slowing down, calming your thoughts, and coming home to yourself.

However, despite yoga's popularity, very few people actually know and experience the full richness of the practice. Some choose to go to a studio for a few hours each week and that is enough for them. Other people yearn for something deeper and want to learn more. If you're reading this book, you may be one of these seekers. You may also simply have an interest in yoga that you are yet to explore!

I'll guide you along the path of yoga, covering everything from where it all started and the ancient yogic philosophies to some foundational poses, breathing techniques, locks, and the basics of sequencing. You'll learn how to put together your own series of poses and how to breathe properly as you move through these sequences. We'll end this book with a guided visualization that you can use in your meditation at the end of each practice.

I hope that *The Yoga Habit* will be like a faithful friend on your yoga adventure. If you apply all you learn, you will inevitably feel more comfortable in your body and feel the positive effects ripple into every area of your life. Ultimately, yoga is about being the best possible version of yourself and feeling good and well. Laughter Yoga (Gendry, 2012) incorporates a song that highlights just the kind of energy I would like to share throughout this book. Let's take a look at the lyrics as a starting point.

"Every little cell in my body is happy.

Every little cell in my body is well.

Feel so good.

Feel so well.

Every little cell in my body is well."

Now, let's get started on your yoga journey!

Chapter 1:

What Is Yoga?

What most of us know of yoga involves the practice of combining various poses or body postures in a sequence, and combining it with controlled breathing. Some say it's a way of stretching stiff muscles, or a way to wind down after a hard day. We carry our mats into a studio, exercise our body, and leave an hour later.

The true essence of yoga, however, is much deeper.

The word *yoga* comes from the Sanskrit term *yuj* which means "union" or "to join" (Living, 2018). Yoga is a spiritual discipline that aims to unite an individual with divine or universal consciousness. It is also a powerful way to achieve harmony between your mind and body, and feel at one with nature and those around you. It's a practice that brings you home to yourself and aligns your body, your mind, and the energy you hold in your entire being.

Yoga moves way beyond poses on the mat and a few breathing techniques. In fact, as we'll soon see, this is

3

only a small part of yoga. Yoga began as an entire way of being. For many, it is a lifestyle and a means of personal transformation. Ancient yogis adhered strictly to the various practices of yoga to achieve liberation and enlightenment.

Maharishi Patanjali based his yoga sutras on ancient sacred texts such as the Rigveda. The Rigveda was written around 8 to 10 thousand years ago and classical yoga forms part of this rich Vedic literature. Approximately 5,000 years ago, Patanjali compiled the Yoga Sutras within which he proposed eight limbs or aspects of yoga (*A Brief History of Yoga*, 2020). Postures and breathwork make up only two of these eight essential components of the practice. It just goes to show—yoga is so much more than we first realized.

Let's go deeper, shall we?

The Eight Limbs of Yoga

Pantanjali's Yoga Sutras speak about the eightfold path to enlightenment. This path is referred to as *ashtanga*, which translated means "eight limbs."

These are essentially eight steps or guidelines on how to live a purposeful life that will result in the soul's liberation. They include all aspects of moral and ethical conduct and self-discipline, and acknowledge both physical and spiritual aspects of our nature.

A true yoga practitioner doesn't just practice the poses, but tries to live by all eight limbs. Let's take a closer look at what each of them involves.

1. Restraints (Yamas)

The *yamas* are ethical standards by which we should live. They provide us with a sense of integrity and focus on our individual behavior and how we conduct ourselves. The yamas are universal practices and relate to how we treat others. They are principles we should align ourselves with and adhere to as much as possible.

There are five different yamas:

Ahimsa, which means non-violence.

Satya, which means honesty and truthfulness.

Asteya, which is non-stealing.

Brahmacharya, which means using your energy correctly.

Aparigraha, which means non-covetousness.

2. Self-Discipline (Niyamas)

The second limb includes the *niyamas* which have to do with spiritual observances and self-discipline. Examples of niyamas in practice include having a daily shower, doing self-inquiry and reflection, and developing a meditation practice.

These are the five niyamas:

Saucha, which means cleanliness.

Santosha, which means contentment despite circumstance.

Tapas refers to heat and spiritual austerities (burning away of desire).

Svadhyaya is the study of sacred scriptures and self-reflection.

Isvara pranidhana is a complete surrender to God.

3. Poses (Asanas)

The third limb includes the *asanas* (poses) which are the yoga postures you perform on your mat. This is what most of us have come to know as yoga. In ancient yogic philosophy, the body is considered a temple of the spirit. Taking care of the body is a sacred practice. By practicing asanas, you will develop a strong habit of discipline, improve your concentration, and through these attributes, be more successful with meditation.

4. Breath Control (Pranayama)

Pranayama, or "breath control" is the fourth limb of yoga. Breathing techniques are designed to master the respiratory process and, through this control, connect the breath, mind, body, and emotions. You can practice breathing control (which we will cover in great detail later on) as an isolated modality, or you can include it as part of your physical yoga practice.

You may have noticed that the first four parts of Patanjali's eight limbs have concentrated on refining your personality, gaining control over your body, and developing an astute energetic awareness. This is all preparation for the next four limbs which involve mastering the senses, fluctuations of the mind, and gaining a higher state of consciousness or being.

5. Sensory Withdrawal (Pratyahara)

The fifth limb is known as *pratyahara*, which is sensory withdrawal and transcendence. This involves making a conscious effort to pull your awareness from the external world and distractions. By maintaining this inward focus and drawing our attention away from our senses, and in a way detaching from them, we are able to take a keen look at ourselves. This introspection allows us to take note of our cravings and habits that may be detrimental to our health and that may be interfering with our spiritual growth.

This sense withdrawal prepares us for the next limb of yoga, which involves the focusing of our thoughts and developing advanced levels of concentration.

6. Concentration (Dharana)

Dharana means concentration. During the process of pratyahara, you absolve yourself from outside distraction. Through dharana, you are able to deal with distraction within your own mind. Concentration precedes meditation and involves learning to slow down our thoughts by focusing on a single mental or physical object. This is called *drishti*—a focused gaze or concentration. What you choose to focus on can be an energetic center in the body, a photograph of a spiritual influence, or perhaps the repetition of a mantra or sound.

As the limbs build on each other, you may start to notice the intelligence of the evolution in the practice of yoga. We start with harnessing our focus in the poses (asanas), controlling our breath and the energies in our body, and then withdrawing our senses, and now learning to take control of our thoughts and attention spans. The more we are able to expand and extend these periods of concentration, the better prepared we will be for meditation.

7. Meditation (Dhyana)

The seventh limb of ashtanga yoga is *dhyana*, or meditation. This is an uninterrupted flow of concentration and focused contemplation. There is a distinct difference between concentration (dharana) and meditation, even though they may appear very similar.

Dharana is the practice of a single point of focus and attention. Dhyana, on the other hand, is about being in a state of awareness with no focus at all. The mind is quiet and produces little to no thoughts. It takes a remarkable sense of stamina to reach this point, and that is why it is important to move through all the stages patiently. Yoga is a process and a journey. It's not about the perfect Instagram pose or a sublime state of consciousness–it's about the evolution into the very best person we can be.

8. Bliss (Samadhi)

This eighth and final limb is described by Patanjali as *samadhi* (a state of ecstasy and bliss). The yoga practitioner, through meditation, merges with their point of focus and transcends the self completely. There is an experience of divine connection and oneness with the universe and everything around you. There is a sacred sense of interconnectedness and a sublime sense of peace. This state of transcendence, or enlightenment, is the ultimate goal of yoga.

Chapter 2:

Benefits of Yoga

As you now know, yoga is about so much more than doing a few poses and potentially working up a sweat in a studio. Yoga is a journey of self-development and overall improvement. There are hundreds of documented benefits of the practice, but I'll mention the 50 most important ones here (yes you read that right—50!).

1. Creates Incredible Flexibility

This is one of the benefits you'll notice after just a few weeks of doing yoga. Many people start off practicing yoga not even able to touch their toes, then within a few months, their palms are flat on the floor. There is a gradual loosening and lengthening of muscles with consistent practice. This increased flexibility isn't just great for pretzel moves; it also reduces nagging aches and pains. Tight hips, for instance, strain the knee joint because the leg's alignment is affected. Tight hamstrings affect the lumbar spine and this can cause lower back pain. Inflexible muscles and ligaments result in poor posture. Regular yoga makes your whole body straighter, stronger, and yes—more bendy.

2. Develops Muscle Strength

Strong muscles look toned and sculpted while protecting us from conditions such as arthritis and back pain. Balancing strength with flexibility in yoga is much more effective for overall well-being than just pumping weights at the gym.

You'll find that over time, you'll be able to hold strength-building poses like Plank Pose for longer and longer periods. Certain standing poses (e.g. Warrior II) and inversions (e.g. Crow Pose) challenge your body's muscles to lift and move the weight of your body. Your muscles respond by stretching and tearing slightly, which in turn grows new muscle fibers. This makes them thicker, more defined, and stronger. This extends way beyond the mat. You'll also be able to lift heavier grocery bags (and those hefty bags of dog food), carry your children for longer, and lug your suitcases across an airport. It may sound silly, but these small acts of independence make you feel good!

3. Improves Your Posture

Poor alignment not only makes your back ache and your muscles overcompensate, but it also leads to fatigue. Your joints will eventually start to suffer and as you slump, your body reacts by flattening the normal curves of your back. This can result in pain and degenerative arthritis. Yoga corrects your posture and realigns your muscles.

4. Prevents Degeneration of Cartilage and Joints

When you practice yoga, your joints move through their full range of motion. This helps prevent degenerative arthritis because it warms up areas of cartilage that usually aren't moving. As you move through different poses, you squeeze and release cartilage. The cartilage around your joints behaves like a sponge. It receives nutrients when its fluid is squeezed out and a new, rich supply is soaked up. Neglected cartilage can eventually wear out and become thin and brittle. This exposes the underlying bone and in turn, rubs against other bones in the joint area, creating pain and swelling.

5. Protects Your Spine's Disks

The disks between your vertebrae act as shock absorbers. These can herniate and compress your nerves if they aren't given the movement and attention they need. These spinal disks crave motion because this is how nutrients are absorbed in the area. This is why backbends, forward bends, and twists are so good for your back. They keep your disks supple and flexible, filled with the goodness they need, and positioned properly.

6. Improves Your Bone Density

Weight-bearing exercises strengthen your bones and help to prevent osteoporosis. This is also true if you're using your own body weight, as you do in yoga (McCall, 2007). Poses like Downward Facing Dog and Upward Facing Dog, for example, help strengthen your arm bones (these are specifically vulnerable to osteoporotic fractures). As yoga decreases the amount of the stress hormone, cortisol, your bone's density is improved and the balance of calcium in your skeleton is maintained (McCall, 2007).

7. Increases Blood Flow and Improves Circulation

Yoga gets your heart pumping and your blood flowing. The various poses and relaxation techniques improve circulation, particularly in your hands and feet. Oxygen fills your cells and they become healthier and function better as a result.

In twisting poses, your internal organs are massaged. This is believed to wring out venous blood and allow oxygenated blood to flow in as you unwind and open space again (McCall, 2007).

Inversions (such as Headstand, Handstand, and Shoulder Stand) allow venous blood to flow from the legs and pelvis to the heart area. It can then be pumped to the lungs, be filled with oxygen, and as you lower back down, refresh your lower limbs. In this way, inverted poses help to reduce swelling in your legs (such as after a long flight), and also aid in healing heart and kidney issues.

Various yoga practices boost levels of hemoglobin and red blood cells which are responsible for carrying oxygen to your organs and tissues. The improved blood flow also thins the blood and makes platelets less sticky, because clot-promoting proteins in the blood are reduced (McCall, 2007). This decreases the risk of heart attacks and strokes because blood clots are often the culprits here.

8. Drains Your Lymph Glands

As you come in and out of yoga poses, and hold them for a while, you engage and stretch your muscles and shift organs around slightly. This movement increases the drainage of lymph, which is a viscous fluid that is transported through vessels in your body. The lymph is rich in immune cells that fight infection, destroy cancerous cells, and dispose of toxic waste products. This process boosts your immunity and helps prevent disease.

9. Elevates Your Heart Rate

Some forms of yoga are aerobic, and this can lower your risk of heart disease. Even styles of yoga that don't elevate your heart rate can improve cardiovascular conditioning. Research has shown that yoga lowers the resting heart rate, increases endurance, and improves how much oxygen you absorb into your cells. One study even found that simple pranayama (breathwork) exercises allowed practitioners to do more exercise with less oxygen (McCall, 2007).

10. Lowers Your Blood Pressure

Two studies published on people suffering from hypertension in Britain compared the effects of Rest Pose (Corpse Pose) as opposed to simply lying down on a couch. After three months, the people who practiced Corpse Pose had a 26-point drop in systolic blood pressure (top range) and a 15-point drop in diastolic blood pressure (bottom range). In fact, the higher the person's initial blood pressure was, the higher the drop (McCall, 2007). Those on the couch didn't have any positive effects.

The alarming part of high blood pressure is that one-fifth of those who have it don't even realize it (Griffin, 2013). Many also struggle with the side effects of medication, especially if it has been a long-term issue. Yoga combined with meditation can slow the heart rate and activate the relaxation response. This calming effect lowers blood pressure and may even bring it down to normal, safe levels. Researchers at the University of Pennsylvania found that 12 weeks of Iyengar Yoga reduced blood pressure even more effectively than nutrition and weight-loss education (Griffin, 2013).

11. Lowers Your Cortisol Levels

Yoga has been shown to lower cortisol levels (McCall, 2007). When your body goes into crisis or stress mode, your adrenal glands secrete cortisol to temporarily boost your immunity. However, sometimes our body holds onto these high levels of cortisol even after the crisis subsides, and this can have a negative impact on our immune systems.

It's a very delicate balance for the body to maintain. For example, a temporary boost of cortisol can help your long-term memory improve. However, if you have abnormally high levels of cortisol in your system, it not only worsens your memory, but can lead to permanent fluctuations in your brain. As an example, excessive cortisol can exacerbate major depression.

Cortisol extracts calcium from your bones which can make osteoporosis symptoms worse. It also elevates your blood pressure and affects the functioning of insulin. High cortisol levels have been linked to overeating or binging when upset, angry, or stressed (McCall, 2007). These extra calories are stored as fat in the belly area and increase the risk of diabetes and heart disease.

Next time you consider binging, tell yourself you can do it right after your yoga practice. Over time, you may find the overeating falls away.

12. Boosts Your Mood

Consistent yoga practice has been shown to increase serotonin levels and improve feelings of depression. Studies done on meditators revealed that the left prefrontal cortex of the brain showed increased activity, and this is directly linked to feelings of happiness (McCall, 2007).

13. Promotes a Healthy Lifestyle

A regular yoga practice will get your muscles moving and this will naturally burn calories and make you more fit. This isn't the only reason your jeans will feel a bit looser, however. The spiritual, mental, and emotional aspects of yoga may also help you eat more consciously and work on any psychological issues around weight management (such as sugar addiction). Yoga also functions to help prevent injury and is a great foundation for other athletics.

14. Decreases Blood Sugar

Yoga has been shown to decrease blood sugar and low-density lipoprotein (LDL) cholesterol (the "bad" one) and increases high-density lipoprotein (HDL) cholesterol (the "good" one). Researchers have also found that yoga lowers blood sugar in people with diabetes (McCall, 2007). This happens through decreasing levels of cortisol and adrenaline, promoting weight loss, and improving sensitivity to insulin and its effects. If you struggle with diabetes, yoga can be an incredible complement to your regular medication. It will help keep your blood sugar levels down and lower your risk of diabetic complications (including kidney failure and blindness).

Researchers at the University of Pittsburgh School of Medicine discovered that adults at risk for type two diabetes who practiced yoga twice a week for a period of three months showed a significant reduction in diabetic risk factors, such as weight and blood pressure (Griffin, 2013).

15. Helps With Concentration

Yoga helps you keep your mind on the present moment. Meditation and mindful yoga practice improve coordination, reaction time, and memory. You'll likely find that you can solve problems more quickly and recall information more effectively. It's also a fantastic antidote if you struggle with negative thinking, because yoga helps you to ease this distraction and return your attention to the here and now.

16. Promotes Relaxation

Yoga encourages a calm and slow breath, promoting relaxation. This provides a natural shift from the sympathetic nervous system (the stressful "fight or flight" response) to the restorative, calming the parasympathetic nervous system. The practice of yoga lowers your heart rate and slows down your breathing, while also deepening your inhalations and exhalations. This, in turn, decreases your blood pressure and your body naturally relaxes. These benefits can be felt almost instantly when you start going through your poses, and are such a relief after a long, hard day at work.

17. Improves Your Balance and Coordination

Regular yoga sessions increase your proprioception, or the ability to sense what your body is doing and where it is in space. For example, even if you're gazing forward, you'll feel what your lifted leg is doing. This improves your balance and coordination.

Usually, people with bad posture or those who struggle with movement patterns (such as toppling over when bending to reach something) have poor proprioception. This has also been linked to joint problems and back pain. Improving your balance could mean fewer trips and falls. For older folks, this can have a dramatic impact on their independence. For younger people, balancing poses such as Tree Pose can make you feel less wobbly (and not just while you're on your mat).

Don't feel embarrassed if you struggle with your sense of balance. In the beginning, we all wobble or even topple over in balancing poses. It's normal! As kids, our day included activities that tested our balance. We walked on narrow curbs, jumped from rock to rock, rode skateboards, and negotiated branches of trees. As adults, most of us spend our time driving, watching TV, or sitting at a desk. None of these activities challenge our balance. Even standard exercise, such as running or swimming, often doesn't directly help our balance. In yoga, your body learns to stay upright, even as you teeter back and forth. Eventually your feet will become more grounded, and you'll feel firmer in your poses. Balancing poses are an integral part of your asana practice.

18. Positively Influences Your Nervous System

As you advance through your yoga practice, you'll be surprised what you can achieve! Some masters can control their bodies in profound ways, and this is usually through amazing control of their nervous systems. Scientists have monitored yoga masters who could induce crazy heart rhythms, generate specific brain-wave patterns, and could even raise the temperature of their hands by a few degrees (Griffin, 2013). It sounds like science fiction, and yet even the average person can learn to influence their nervous system. For example, you can potentially reduce trouble falling asleep by inducing deep levels of relaxation.

19. Releases Muscle Tension

We all have daily habits that may be contributing to muscular tension. For example, if you hold your phone between your ear and shoulder, or perhaps grip your car's steering wheel very tightly. You may squint when staring at a computer screen or hunch your shoulders at your desk. We do all of this unconsciously, and yet it can have long-lasting effects. This can be experienced through things such as a stiff neck, sore back, muscle fatigue, aching wrists, or even jaw pain. These aches and pains only aggravate stress and a bad mood.

When you do yoga, you soon realize where you're holding tension in your body (this differs from person to person). Some people feel tension in their eyes and only notice when the pain goes away while relaxing in Corpse Pose. Other people tense their neck and shoulders and feel the stiffness (and relief) in Cat/Cow Pose. Yoga is a beautiful way to get to know your body and the unique way you carry tension. This awareness of tension patterns can support you to release them.

20. Deepens Sleep and Relieves Insomnia

Modern life can become incredibly busy and stressful. This has a direct impact on our sleeping patterns. It's not unusual for us to lie awake at night and think about all the concerns of our lives. You may also struggle to fall asleep or battle to wake up in the mornings. This constant stimulation takes its toll on your nervous system. Yoga can bring relief.

Restorative poses, yoga nidra (a form of guided relaxation), Corpse Pose, pranayama (breathing techniques), and various forms of meditation encourage pratyahara. You may recall that this is the inward turning of your senses. Your nervous system gets a break and your body slows down.

The natural effect of these relaxing yogic techniques is better sleep. You'll wake up feeling more refreshed, less exhausted and stressed, and will very likely be a better person to be around! When we're fatigued we can become irritable, frustrated, and snappy.

Yoga poses (asanas) stretch and relax your muscles, helping you to unwind after a long day. Breathing exercises (pranayama) can slow your heart rate and prepare you for a good night's sleep. Regular meditation (especially just before bedtime) can prevent you from getting tangled up in the thoughts that tend to keep you awake. And can help you rest better.

21. Expands Your Lungs

Yoga practices promote breathing through the nose, such as when you use the ocean breath during a yoga class (I will explain exactly how to perform this breathing technique later on). Breathing through your nose filters the air and warms it up. This is important because cold, dry air can trigger asthma attacks in sensitive people and is not as relaxing. Nose-breathing also humidifies the air, removes pollen and other dirt, and is overall a much healthier way of breathing than when you only do so through your mouth.

People who practice yoga regularly take fewer, deeper breaths. This is not only calming, but also much more efficient.

22. Eases Digestive Issues

Our digestive tract is often the first indicator of imbalance in our bodies. It is sensitive to stress and you may suffer from digestive issues such as irritable bowel syndrome (IBS), constipation, acid reflux, or even more serious conditions such as ulcers.

Yoga eases these types of symptoms and promotes active digestion. As you massage your organs, such as through deep twists, you help to facilitate movement of food and waste.

Naturally, the stress-relieving properties of yoga also decrease the risk of ulcers and other painful digestive problems.

23. Boosts Your Immunity

Yoga poses and breathing techniques positively affect your immune system, but meditation comes out on top in this area. Meditation can help prevent you from getting sick, and can also calm inflammatory responses. Both yoga and meditation help boost the immune system through stress reduction, as well as through inclining you towards healthier habits in general.

24. Decreases Your Stress

The various practices of yoga slow down the fluctuations in your mind and thoughts. When you're focusing on the current moment while in Warrior I, you're not thinking about your frustrating day or the argument you had earlier. As you try to balance and breathe deeply in Triangle Pose, you forget about your usual fears and anxieties. Just an hour of practice can reduce your overall levels of stress quite dramatically.

Quieting your mind can also alleviate migraines and lower your blood pressure, bringing your body back to a state of calm. This may have a direct impact on your longevity and quality of life.

25. Enhances Your Self-Esteem

You may suffer from feelings of self-doubt or low self-esteem. Some people respond to this in a negative way in order to cope. This can manifest in various ways, such as through drug or alcohol addiction, overeating, working too hard, or not taking care of yourself in general.

Yoga is a positive modality and even a type of therapy in some cases. It teaches you that you are part of a greater whole and connected with every living thing. You'll begin to sense your value and that you're worthwhile, simply because you have breath.

As you incorporate the various yogic philosophies and teachings into your life, you'll learn to self-examine yourself more deeply and you'll realize that you reflect aspects of the Divine. You are an incredible human being, and yoga helps you see this more clearly.

Yoga gives us a sense that we are all part of something bigger and that we each have something valuable to offer the world. We feel more gratitude, empathy, and forgiveness (to others and ourselves), and our belief in ourselves grows the more we practice.

26. Eases Your Aches and Pains

Regularly practicing yoga can ease your pain (such as arthritis, back pain, carpal tunnel syndrome, fibromyalgia, and other chronic conditions). Relieving your pain not only helps you on a physical level, but also improves your mood, inspires you to live a more active life, and can even help you cut back on pain-reducing medication.

27. Builds Inner Strength and Resolve

This is perhaps one of the greatest strengths of yoga. It helps us make difficult decisions and embrace the changes that we need to make. You may recall the word *tapas* from when we spoke about the eight limbs of yoga. *Tapas* means "heat," literally the fire or discipline that builds from within and gets us onto our mat each day. This inner resolve fuels our confidence beyond the mat too.

If you're stuck in your ways, the cultivation of this heat or inner resolve will help you overcome your inertia. When you practice yoga regularly (and this in itself takes heated discipline), you naturally start to eat better, exercise more regularly, and may even quit bad habits such as smoking (despite multiple previous attempts to do so in the past).

To some of us, yoga truly is a miracle!

28. Connects you With Extraordinary Teachers

If you practice yoga at a studio, or one-on-one with a teacher, and possibly even online, you may have noticed that you have a favorite instructor or two. Good yoga teachers can make all the difference to your progress in yoga and with your health and self-development.

Yoga instructors are not there to simply guide you through the postures and give you a cool playlist. Teachers can adjust your poses, gauge when you can go deeper and guide you there physically, know when to back off and let your body use its own wisdom, and may even push you out of your comfort zone (that first time in a Headstand can be scary!).

Good yoga teachers also know how to guide you through a meditation or yoga nidra practice and help you relax in Corpse Pose at the end of class. Your practice can be personalized and you'll likely grow and advance more steadily in your yoga journey through these types of guiding relationships.

29. Decreases Your Need for Medication

Some of us have medicine cabinets that would overwhelm a pharmacist. We have asthma inhalers, pills for high blood pressure, tablets for menstrual pain, insulin injections, and/or mood disorder stabilizers.

Studies have shown that people with asthma, high blood pressure, type two diabetes, and obsessive-compulsive disorder can reduce their dosages of medications if they practice yoga regularly (Griffin, 2013). Some people even wean themselves off drugs entirely!

Lower dosages mean fewer side effects, lower risk of drug interactions, and reduced medical expenses.

30. Improves Your Awareness

Meditation and yoga build self-awareness. If you're aware, you're more likely to break free from toxic emotions, such as anger. Chronic aggression and hostility are linked to heart disease, especially when coupled with diabetes, smoking, and high cholesterol (Griffin, 2013).

Yoga seems to reduce anger through increasing positive emotions for people suffering from hypertension, such as compassion and interconnection. As we've spoken about before, yoga calms the mind and nervous system, increases your ability to step back from what is happening in your life, and helps us remain steady. Even if you're faced with unsettling news, you'll be equipped to react more rationally. Your behavior becomes more thoughtful and compassionate.

31. Strengthens Your Relationships

A regular yoga practice helps to propagate friendliness, compassion, and acceptance. Love and empathy heal. Friends, family, and community make a tremendous difference to your mental well-being. The yoga community often becomes like family, and the people you spend time with in the studio may turn into lifelong friends.

Yogic philosophy teaches us to avoid harming others, to tell the truth, and to take only what we need. These aspects alone strengthen our relationships dramatically.

32. Chanting and Sound Clear Your Sinuses

Chanting—even if it's just the sound of "om" at the beginning of class, is incredibly soothing. Chanting prolongs our exhalations which shifts the balance of our nervous system. It's also a powerful emotional experience, and the physical vibrations of the sound can be healing. Humming sounds, as performed in the Brahmari breath (which we will cover in detail later), can open the sinuses and bring our attention inward.

33. Visualization can Promote Healing

At the end of practice, it is common to spend a few minutes relaxing and meditating. If you are able to contemplate an image in your mind's eye, you can create change in your physical body as well (Griffin, 2013). For example, guided imagery during yoga nidra can reduce pain (it's especially useful for headaches) and improve the quality of life for people who are struggling with chronic pain (such as those with cancer). Visualization sets the tone for what is possible.

34. Certain Yogic Practices Ease Allergies

Some types of yoga incorporate *kriyas* into their practices. *Kriyas* are cleansing techniques and include multiple practices, such as rapid breathing exercises, internal cleansing of the intestines, and *jala neti* (gentle cleansing of the nasal passages with salt water). This may sound a bit unusual, but it removes pollen and viruses and prevents mucus from building up. This drains the sinuses and eases the effects of allergies.

35. Builds a Life of Service

The part of yoga that is dedicated to the service of others is called *karma* yoga. It is an integral aspect of ancient yogic philosophy. Service brings meaning to our lives, as helping others immediately makes us feel better, and this has an impact on our health. You may wish to start volunteering in your community toward a cause that is close to your heart.

36. Encourages Self-Care and Self-Love

Although yoga can certainly be about (and should include) service to others, the entire practice is actually about developing yourself and growing towards enlightenment and personal freedom. What you do for yourself genuinely matters.

Yoga provides you with the tools to change your life. You should start to feel better about yourself the more you practice. The more committed you are, the more you benefit.

You take personal responsibility for your own care and learn to put yourself first. You learn that you have the power within you to bring about remarkable change, and that there is always hope. Hope is healing and giving this gift to yourself is the ultimate act of self-care.

37. Strengthens Your Connections

Yoga improves your health in so many ways and they often overlap (as you may have noticed as you've been reading). It's as if there is a ripple effect when you practice. One positive benefit results in the next, and so on.

For example, if you change your posture, your breathing automatically changes as well. When our breathing changes (such as when you take deeper, longer breaths) you make subtle shifts in your nervous system.

This is what yoga teaches us. Everything is connected. Your wrist is connected to your elbow and your elbow is connected to your shoulder. Your family is connected to your community and your community is connected to the world. This interconnectedness is fundamental to yoga. At the heart of it all, you realize that you are not alone and that every part of you is connected on some level to every living thing.

38. Uses the Power of Affirmations

The power of belief is incredible. If you think you will get better, you probably will. Believing that you will be able to get into a backbend makes all the difference. This is where affirmations and mantras become so powerful, as is setting an intention at the start of class.

In the yoga sequences later on in this book, I include some affirmations that you can say throughout your practice. By repeating these phrases over and over again as your body moves, you slowly start to believe them.

39. Relieves Pain

Yoga doesn't just help with normal aches and pains, it even shows promise as a treatment for severe and chronic pain. There was a study conducted in Germany with groups of people suffering from chronic neck pain that compared Iyengar Yoga with a normal self-care exercise program. They discovered that yoga reduced pain scores by more than 50 percent (Griffin, 2013).

Rheumatoid arthritis is a debilitating autoimmune disorder where the body attacks the lining of the joints. It is an incredibly painful disease. Researchers at the University of California, Los Angeles studied young women suffering from this disorder and found that half of them who took part in a yoga program reported improvements in their levels of pain and also showed a decrease in their associated anxiety and depression (Griffin, 2013).

40. Anyone can do it

There is no discrimination when it comes to yoga. It doesn't matter if you're overweight and inactive, or if you have an injury or an illness. Yoga is accessible for anyone at any level.

Kim Innes, a Kundalini Yoga teacher and associate professor at the University of Virginia, did research on beginner yogis in various studies. She says, "Even those who thought they 'could not do yoga,' noted benefits after the first session. My belief is that once people are exposed to gentle yoga practice with an experienced yoga therapist, they will likely become hooked very quickly" (Griffin, 2013).

41. Eases Depression

Depression has become a silent killer, and especially as a result of the global COVID-19 pandemic, which is still impacting the human community as I write this, more and more people are admitting they are struggling. New research has explored the ways in which yoga can benefit this worldwide mental health problem.

One of the main problems with depression is constant rumination and negative thoughts. It's not only seated meditation that can slow this thinking down. Mindful progression through yoga poses has a similar effect. When you're considering which way your hips are facing or are feeling your thighs burning while doing Chair Pose, you're not thinking about your daily stresses. You're focused on being mindful in the moment, and it's all about where you focus your attention.

Modern technologies such as functional MRI screenings are now proving what ancient yoga masters have known all along: Yoga affects the brain. We become less reactive and emotionally explosive through this practice, as can be seen in scans taken of long-term yoga practitioners' brains.

Yoga makes you emotionally resilient and more positive. It helps you tackle life's problems instead of letting them overwhelm you. It won't necessarily happen after doing one Downward Facing Dog, but a regular, daily practice will certainly have an impact on your moods.

42. Improves Focus

Yoga poses, breathing techniques, and meditation fine-tune your attention and focus. You learn to sync your breath with movement and pick up on the subtle movements inside and throughout your body. You let go of thoughts and bring your mind toward a positive affirmation. This intense concentration helps your brain function better overall. Research has shown that after doing 20 minutes of yoga, subjects completed a set of mental challenges faster and more accurately than they did after a quick run (Griffin, 2013).

43. Results in Better Sex

Yoga has been proven to improve several areas of sexuality including desire, orgasm, and overall satisfaction (Griffin, 2013). It increases blood flow and circulation, including to the erogenous regions. It also makes you more in tune with your own body, making you feel better about yourself. Plus, if we're being really honest, flexibility and stamina must surely play a role too!

44. Slows Down Inflammation

Inflammation is your body's way of healing itself. For example, if you sprain your ankle, the swelling will help immobilize the joint so that you don't hurt yourself further. However, sometimes inflammation kicks into overdrive and the body turns on itself. People who suffer from autoimmune disorders, for instance, have an excessive inflammatory response. Their body cannot tell the difference between a threat (such as a virus) and its own tissue, so it literally starts to attack itself.

This type of damaging inflammation is often triggered by stress. People who practice yoga regularly have lower blood levels of inflammation-promoting immune cells than those who don't (Griffin, 2013). Seasoned yoga practitioners respond differently to stress (compared to those who never practice yoga) and have lower levels of disease-causing inflammation.

45. Has an Anti-Aging Effect

Yoga and meditation have been associated with cellular changes that affect how the body ages (Griffin, 2013). Our cells include structures called telomeres. These little guys are bits of DNA at the end of chromosomes. Every time a cell divides, the telomeres get shorter and shorter. If they get too short, the cells can't divide anymore, and they die (which is a key part of our bodies aging). Yoga helps to preserve the length of these telomeres.

A study was done on men with prostate cancer who did yoga for one hour a day, six days a week. They showed a 30 percent increase of activity in a key enzyme called telomerase (which preserves telomeres at the tips of our DNA). In a similar research study, a group of stressed caregivers took part in a program that combined meditation, yoga and chanting. They showed a 39 percent increase in telomerase activity compared with another group who only listened to music (Griffin, 2013).

It may not stop you from getting gray hair, but yoga will certainly help ease stiff joints, slow down disease, and make you feel and look younger.

46. Strengthens Your Spine

It has been well documented that yoga helps ease back pain. The main reason is that yoga postures bring our bodies back into alignment, and muscles that have overcompensated for our poor posture and slouching behavior at our desks become stretched and soothed. Even just doing a few rounds of Standing Forward Folds and an easy backbend such as Bridge Pose will go a long way in strengthening your spine.

47. Maintains a Healthy Heart

Heart disease is the number one cause of death in men and women in the United States. It is usually caused by high blood pressure, high cholesterol, high blood sugar, and an inactive lifestyle. As you now know, all of these conditions are positively impacted by yoga.

In a study conducted by researchers at the University of Kansas Medical Center, people who took part in two sessions of yoga a week (which included breathing techniques and asana practice) had a dramatic reduction in the frequency of atrial fibrillation episodes (Griffin,

2013). Atrial fibrillation is a disorder that affects the rhythm of the heart and increases the risk of heart failure and strokes. Doing yoga can reduce these risks and support you to have a healthy heart.

48. Strengthens Your Joints

Yoga takes your joints through their entire range of motion. This keeps them lubricated and moving freely. A common complaint, for instance, is tight hips. Regular inclusion of poses such as Warrior II and Tree Pose can help open your hips and lengthen the muscles around your hip joints, making them stronger and more stable.

49. Soothes Menopausal Symptoms

The various symptoms of menopause can be very frustrating, and in some cases, even debilitating. Hot flashes, mood swings, and sleep disturbances are all eased by regular yoga practice. For example, inversions provide relief from anxiety and irritability which are common during hormonal fluctuations. However, it's important to use supported and restorative poses for the best results. An unsupported Headstand, for example, may worsen hot flashes, while a slightly modified inversion (such as Bridge Pose supported with bolsters) will provide the benefits you are after.

50. Makes you Feel Good

This is yoga in a nutshell: It makes you feel good and more alive. Exercise is linked with higher levels of a brain chemical known as gamma-aminobutyric acid (GABA) which is linked with positive mood and a sense of well-being (Griffin, 2013). Looking great in a smaller jean size is another fantastic mood-booster!

Now that you have a thorough understanding of what yoga is, you may be incredibly keen to start practicing yourself! Before we get into the poses and different yoga techniques, you will need to invest in a good yoga mat and perhaps a few other props. We'll look at these in more detail in the next chapter.

Chapter 3:

Props and Equipment

Fortunately with yoga, you really don't need a lot to get started. You will have to invest in a decent yoga mat, and perhaps a block or two. Let's dive into all the goodies available, then you can decide what you need and take it from there.

Choosing a Good Yoga Mat

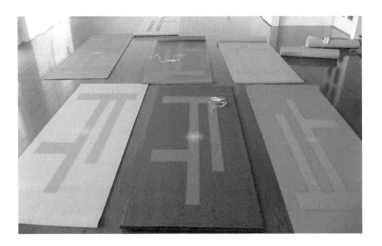

Your yoga mat is the most important investment in your yoga journey. There are many different types to choose from, and you may be overwhelmed with making a decision. I'll walk you through the different aspects to consider when choosing a mat, but in the end, it remains a very personal decision. Your lifestyle and unique preferences will help guide you.

Thickness

A standard yoga mat is usually ⅛ inch thick, but this can be too thin for some people. If you're thin and bony, or if you struggle with knee pain, this may not be thick enough. For example, when you're in Bow Pose, your hip bones will press against the floor and, if your mat doesn't offer enough support, it may hurt you. You may wish to invest in a thicker mat (¼ inch thick).

However, you also need to keep in mind that thicker mats are more spongy and can make balancing poses (such as Tree Pose) more challenging. In addition, the extra cushioning makes the mat bulky and heavier, and thus more difficult to carry. Before investing in a thicker mat, consider what your yoga goals are and what is best suited to your body's needs.

Texture

There are a range of different textures to choose from. You can go for sticky, smooth, velvety, or even cork.

Smooth mats can be fantastic because some of them give you the "sticky" feel. This helps you grip the mat and prevents you from sliding around. For example, in Downward Facing Dog, if a mat is too smooth and slippery, your hands and feet can slide and make you lose your balance. If you choose a smooth mat, make sure it has good traction, because a slippery one can potentially be dangerous.

Polyvinyl chloride (PVC) mats that are completely smooth are not good choices if you're going to be doing Vinyasa or Ashtanga yoga which requires fast, powerful movements. They're also not designed for hot yoga, because your sweat on the smooth surface will create a very slippery experience.

Natural rubber mats are smooth but more "sticky" and they don't absorb sweat as much as a textured mat (which may soon start smelling).

Mats with textured patterns provide natural grip and are made from cotton or jute. Some rubber mats also come with a suede-like texture that is wonderful for gentle types of yoga, such as Yin Yoga.

Length

Your mat needs to be long enough to support your whole body when you lie down in Savasana (Rest Pose). Standard yoga mats are about 68 inches long, so if you're taller than this you should invest in an extra-long mat.

Some mats are wider than average, which is not only great if you need the extra space to accommodate your body size, but also for poses that involve lying on your back and twisting over to one side.

Keep in mind that longer and wider mats are heavier and bulkier. There are also fewer mat bags made for longer and wider mats, although manufacturers are also realizing that these are becoming more popular.

Yoga Clothes

Any clothing you can move around in can work fine for yoga. However, as you get into yoga, you likely will want designated clothes for wearing during practice time. The benefit of clothes designed specifically for yoga is that they are streamlined and simple in their form, making them less disruptive, or even supportive, to your practice. Most yogis feel that the clothes you can forget about while practicing, leaving you to focus on presence in the practice unencumbered, are the best choice.

For women, a tight-fitting tank top with a built-in shelf-bra often works well. Some yoginis like to wear a crop top. It is really a matter of personal preference, both in terms of style and function. If you need a lot of chest support, look for a tank top with a higher neckline, so that you stay supported even when you are bending forward or upside down.

Yoga pants come in all sorts of styles; the main difference you will find is how loose or tight-fitting they are. This again is a matter of personal preference in terms of style and function. Looser pants with a wider bottom can feel more comfortable, but can also get in the way or be distracting for some yoga practitioners. Tighter-fitting leggings can be easier to totally forget while you focus on practice, as long as they don't feel too restrictive, especially at the knees. Some women like to wear skin-hugging shorts.

For men, you can wear any athletic shorts or pants that suit you for moves where you may be upside-down or stretching your leg way out to the side or even up towards your head. For this reason, some men wear tight-fitting leggings or shorts, and a form-fitting tank top or no shirt. You can, of course, buy clothes specifically designed for men doing yoga. Make sure whatever you wear is comfortable and keeps your privates private. Cut off any bothersome tags.

Ideally, practice in a warm environment, especially for more active forms of yoga. In a warm room, you can be comfortable with your arms bare, which can support you to move into poses with more ease. However, if you prefer a more modest look, that is fine too.

Some yogis like to buy organic cotton yoga clothes, so they don't absorb chemicals when they sweat.

Yoga practice is a time to enjoy your physical experience in your body, so choose clothes that make you feel good. In the end, what feels best to you is the right yoga outfit.

Yoga Props

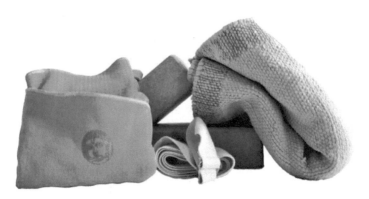

Not all bodies are made to squeeze and struggle their way into each pose. We are all unique and even with years of practice, there may simply be some asanas that your body will never get into without support. This is normal.

While we're building up our strength and extending our range of flexibility (which may be advanced with some muscles and beginner level at others), it's essential to use different types of props. This not only supports us as we gain extra mobility and stamina, but also helps to prevent injury.

Let's take a closer look at the types of yoga props that are available and when and how to use them.

Blankets

A yoga blanket can be used for seated poses, to add cushion and comfort. Some blankets have grip on one side. They come in varying styles and thicknesses.

Bolsters

Using a bolster is most common in restorative yoga classes or poses and is widely used in Yin Yoga. It is usually a long, firm, and narrow pillow shaped like a cylinder or rectangle. It's incredibly supportive and comforting when spending a long time in a particular pose, or while doing deep breathing exercises. They are particularly useful if you are recovering from an injury, are pregnant, or get tired easily. For example, if you have lower back pain, you can place a bolster underneath your knees when you lie down in Corpse Pose.

It's also a wonderful addition to Child's Pose. You simply place it between your legs before you fold over your thighs. Another great example is Legs Up The Wall Pose. Here you place the bolster under your pelvis and allow your legs to lean straight against a wall. Both are beautiful restorative poses.

We'll cover all the necessary poses that a beginner needs to know later on in this book, so don't worry if a certain pose name is unfamiliar to you right now.

Blocks

Yoga blocks are usually made of foam, bamboo, wood, or cork. You can use a block as an extension of your arm, such as when you aren't able to reach the floor in a pose like Half Moon. Blocks can also be used to support the back, head, and hips in floor-based postures.

Blocks "bring the floor closer" to your body and shorten the distance you need to lean, bend, and stretch. It supports your range of motion so that you can come into proper alignment without having to stretch and extend beyond your capability.

If you're struggling with an injury or physical limitation, a block can be a fantastic support. Blocks are particularly useful when holding poses for long periods of time. For example, when kneeling in meditation you can place a block between your legs for support.

Depending on how you place the block, you can use low, medium, or high positions. This makes them extremely versatile. Keep one or two next to your mat each time you practice. You never know when they'll come in handy.

Straps

Yoga straps have so many benefits for all, from beginners all the way through to advanced practitioners. If you don't have a strap, you can use a belt or non-stretchy scarf. Yoga straps can also serve the same purpose as an exercise band because they provide resistance when buckled or knotted. The primary functions of a yoga strap are to correct alignment, deepen stretches, and advance your practice.

Let's take a look at each of these functions in detail.

Correct Alignment

It's all too tempting to try and force yourself into a pose that your body isn't ready for yet. It may look cool, but sadly misalignment comes at a high price. A rounded back and muscles forced into positions can result in injury. Even if you manage to get your body into a pose, if you are out of alignment, there is no point.

A yoga strap allows you to practice a pose and feel what it feels like in proper alignment, but without injuring yourself.

Here's an example: Chaturanga (Low Plank)

This is a really challenging pose, and it takes a while to build up your strength to perform it properly. Low Plank requires upper body strength and, to make the pose easier, some people automatically splay their elbows out. Using a strap keeps your arms tucked against your ribs and allows you to build the strength you need to perform this pose properly.

We'll go into this pose step-by-step later on, but here is a brief idea of how a strap can help you.

1. Place your strap above the elbows and set it to shoulder width (you can do this with the buckle it comes with or simply tie a firm knot). Keep the strap taut so that your elbows don't collapse outward in the pose.

2. From Plank Pose (we'll cover this one later too), shift forward and move downwards until your chest touches the strap. This is how a Low Plank feels!

Deepen Stretches

Yoga straps make it possible for you to deepen stretches such as Seated Forward Folds (yup, we'll definitely cover this one!). Straps provide resistance so that you can go deeper into a pose while maintaining your alignment. Eventually, once you've built up your flexibility, you won't need it anymore.

Here's an example: Seated Forward Fold

This is a great hamstring stretch, but people often round their backs while trying to fold all the way forward to reach their toes. Using a strap provides resistance that prevents your back from hunching over, and this allows a deeper stretch in your hamstrings.

1. Sit on your mat and place the strap under the balls of your feet.

2. Straighten your legs and flex your feet. Now exhale and fold, keeping your spine straight, while pulling the strap towards you. Feels good, right?

Another way that straps can assist with deepening a stretch is in binds. There are variations to certain poses, such as Extended Side Angle and Reverse Warrior, where your hands come behind your back and clasp each other. The aim is to open the chest and get a deeper stretch. However, a common mistake is going into this bind too soon and losing alignment as your body compensates.

Using a strap makes it possible for you to go into the bind without having to have the flexibility of your hands reaching each other. The yoga strap provides the length you need, and as you advance, you can walk your hands closer and closer along the strap. Eventually, your fingers will touch!

Here's an example: Extended Side Angle Bind

1. Begin in Warrior II pose (of course, we'll cover this later) with your right knee bent.

2. Bring your right hand down to the inside of your right foot and lift your left arm up (holding the strap), opening your chest.

3. Bend your right arm to reach under your right thigh and move your left hand behind your back, dangling the strap towards your right hand.

4. Reach for the strap with your right hand and then "walk" your way up the strap until you meet your

resistance point. This opens your chest even more.

Lengthen Muscles

Straps allow you to master poses quicker and also allow you to feel a pose even if you can't fully get into it yet. For example, many people battle to have their feet reach their head in King Pigeon Pose, but when you use a strap you will know how your hips and arms should be aligned. You can move the strap closer and closer until your feet eventually touch your head. All the while you're lengthening the muscles you need in order to achieve the pose without a prop later on.

Here are two examples of where you can use a strap to advance your poses. I'll use poses that we will cover in more detail later.

Tree Pose

This is a balancing posture that can be difficult in the beginning, especially if you have tight hips. As you don't want your foot resting on your knee, a yoga strap can provide the support you need to reach your thigh by opening your hip and guiding your foot upwards. It also provides resistance which helps with balancing.

1. Start from a standing position and wrap your strap around your left foot.

2. Shift your weight to the right foot and lift your left leg up, bending it towards your chest.

3. Rest your left foot on your right inner thigh by guiding it with the strap. Repeat on the other side.

Warrior III

Warrior III requires a fair amount of balance and can be challenging for beginners. It involves hinging forward while standing on one leg. Using a yoga strap provides traction and support so that you can focus on your alignment without toppling over.

1. Start in a standing position and hook the strap under your left foot, and then grab it with your hands behind your back.

2. Shift your weight onto your right leg and hinge forward, firmly holding the strap, until your torso is in line with your left leg. Your leg should be at a 90-degree angle to the floor.

3. Flex your toes and keep pulling the strap to maintain your balance.

There are other props you can use such as towels (to absorb sweat and prevent slipping in hot yoga classes), blankets (to keep you warm in Corpse Pose), and eye pillows (for that extra darkness and inward-focus when meditating).

Once you have your basic equipment (and you truly only need a yoga mat to get started), you're ready to learn some poses. We'll do that in the next chapter!

Chapter 4:

Time, Frequency, and Temperature

What time of day is best for practicing yoga?

Traditionally, yoga has most often been practiced first thing in the morning, before or with the rising sun. It is considered best to practice yoga on an empty stomach. Late afternoon or early evening can also be a good time, provided you have not eaten recently.

If you do your yoga late at night, close to bedtime, it may be best to practice a less rigorous form of yoga, especially if you have recently eaten dinner, or if restful activities help you wind down for sleep. Early morning or late afternoon up until dinner time, for most yogis, are good times for more rigorous practice.

There may be other reasons for this suggested timing, including the fact that, for most people, yoga is intended to be either a support for getting your day started or a way to wind down from your workday, household care, and life-building day out in the world.

You may consider taking a day of rest from yoga on the new and full moon days. I also encourage women to take a day off from yoga on the first day of menstruation, and longer if you need.

How often should you practice?

The short answer is whenever you can! Ideally, you engage in your yoga habit at least three days per week. Some yogis practice six days per week, with one day to rest. Others take rest from practice only on the new moon and full moon days. You can also practice regularly once in the morning and again in the evening. Find a good rhythm for your lifestyle and try to stick with it!

What temperature is best for practicing yoga?

Yoga practice supports the body to develop internal heat (tapas). If you join my mailing list, which is linked at the back of this book, I intend to discuss this topic in more detail there. (Along with Yoga for Hands and Feet, and more.) For now, I want to mention that cultivation of internal heat is good for your circulation, as well as your immune system, and may be best developed in the cooler parts of the day.

A warm room can feel good, and it is important that you enjoy your yoga time. I do not personally recommend hot yoga (where the room is purposefully heated like a sauna.) While sweating is certainly good for you, I encourage you to make yoga practice a time to focus on supporting heat from within.

Chapter 5:

Strike a Pose

Now that you know the basics of yoga and what you'll need, it's time to get down to the nitty-gritty. This chapter will outline the foundational poses (asanas) that you need to master and how to do them, step-by-step. I'll also provide modification tips for each one, because if you're a beginner you'll need to gradually build up your strength and flexibility. Fortunately, each pose is easily adapted according to your current practice level.

The Core Vinyasa Flow

In most yoga classes, regardless of style, there will be a familiar series of four poses that are performed in the same sequence. It's sometimes called a basic Vinyasa flow, and is often used to transition between different parts of the class. It is also a key part of Sun Salutations. You'll come to know this sequence well: You move from Plank Pose to Low Plank (also commonly known by its

Sanskrit name, *Chaturanga*), then into Upward Facing Dog, and finally into Downward Facing Dog.

We'll now take a closer look at each of these steps so that you flow with proper alignment and have the correct form throughout.

1. Plank Pose

Alternative name: High plank

Sanskrit name: *Phalakasana*

Associated chakra: Solar plexus (Manipura chakra)

Element: Fire

Closely related poses: Forearm Plank, Low Plank, Side Plank

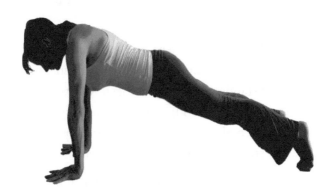

Plank Pose Step-by-Step

1. Start in Tabletop Position, with your wrists directly below your shoulders and your knees in line with your hips. Check the position of your hands. Your fingers should be pointing forwards (your middle fingers parallel to the sides of your mat), and your fingers spread wide. Try to push down through your fingertips and lift your finger joints a smidgen off the mat. This helps create stability in your hands.

2. Press your hands into the floor as if you're pushing the ground away from you. Make sure the insides of your elbows are facing each other so that your arms aren't rotated outwards.

3. Tighten your core by pulling your belly button in towards your spine and up towards your upper back.

4. Extend your legs behind you with your toes tucked (you'll be hovering in plank while "standing" on your toes). Contract your glutes (your rear end), engage your thigh muscles, and keep that core engaged. Your body will be in a straight line from head to heels.

5. Take care not to drop your hips or lift them higher than the line of your body.

6. Relax your neck and gaze at a point on your mat just a few inches in front of your hands.

7. Imagine someone is placing their hand between your shoulder blades and adjust your position so that you are "pushing their hand away." This slight shift will get your shoulders into proper alignment.

8. Without moving your legs, draw them towards each other. It helps to imagine you're holding a block between your thighs and that you need to keep it there. This creates stability in your pose.

Modifications

● You can build your strength by doing Plank Pose with your knees on the floor. Start by getting into full plank and then, while keeping your torso and upper thighs in line, drop your knees to the floor. The list of steps remains exactly the same as above, except you'll be balancing your lower body on your knees instead of your toes, as a way of reducing the weight on your wrists. This helps if you haven't got enough strength in your upper body yet to hold normal Plank Pose.

● If your wrists get sore in plank, you can place a rolled up towel under the heels of your hands. This reduces the angle of the bend in your wrists.

Benefits

● Develops your core strength and stability.

● Strengthens and tones your whole body.

- Prepares your body and mind for other arm balances and inversions.

2. Low Plank

Alternative names: Four-limbed Staff Pose, Four-Limbed Stick Pose, Chaturanga

Sanskrit name: *Chaturanga Dandasana*

Associated chakra: Solar plexus (Manipura chakra)

Element: Fire

Closely related poses: Forearm Plank, Plank Pose, Upward Facing Dog

Low Plank Step-by-Step

1. Starting from Plank Pose, focus on engaging your core and tightening your glutes and thighs so that your body feels like a solid, straight rod.

2. Rock slightly forward so that your shoulders extend beyond your wrists, and your heels are pushing forward over your toes.

3. Keep your gaze slightly ahead of you and your neck long (relaxed and in line with your straight spine).

4. On an exhale, lower your whole body toward the ground, but stop when your elbows graze past your ribs. Your upper arms will be parallel to your mat, with a 90-degree angle in your elbows. It's

important to keep your elbows close against your ribs (not flailing out to the sides).

5. Don't allow your chest and shoulders to dip lower than your elbows (that is going down too low). Your shoulders should be completely parallel to the ground.

6. For an extra challenge in this pose, you can try lowering down from plank with only one foot on your mat, and the other leg raised parallel to the floor.

Modifications

Low Plank requires a lot of strength and is often difficult for beginners to master. While you're building stamina, you can do a "Baby Chaturanga" instead, where you lower your knees to the floor (while maintaining a straight line from your head to your knees).

Benefits

- Strengthens your core, wrists, arms, and legs.

- An excellent preparatory pose for other arm balances such as Crow Pose.

3. Upward Facing Dog

Alternative name: Up Dog

Sanskrit name: *Urdhva Mukha Svanasana*

Associated chakras: Throat (Vishuddha chakra), Heart (Anahata chakra), Solar plexus (Manipura chakra), Sacral (Swadisthana chakra), Root (Muladhara chakra)

Elements: Ether, Air, Fire, Water, Earth

Closely related poses: Bow Pose, Cobra Pose, Downward Facing Dog, Sphinx Pose

Upward Facing Dog Step-by-Step

1. You'll be moving from Low Plank (Chaturanga) into Upward Facing Dog.

2. On an inhale, glide forward as you untuck your toes (the tops of your feet will be pressed against the mat) and straighten your arms.

3. Your shoulders should be directly above your wrists, and your chest drawing forwards through your arms. Your back will naturally curve (this pose is considered a "backbend").

4. Keep your gaze straight ahead or slightly upward.

5. Draw your shoulders away from your ears to ensure you aren't "hanging" in the pose.

6. Your knees and hips should not be touching the mat. Keep your legs and glutes active and engaged as this will help you keep your knees off the ground.

Modifications

You can start by doing Cobra Pose instead, and then as you gain strength in your arms and shoulders, you can progress to Upward Facing Dog. We'll cover Cobra Pose later in this chapter.

Benefits

- Opens the chest and lungs.

- Stretches the whole front side of your body, chest, and intercostal muscles between your ribs.

- Strengthens your wrists, arms, shoulders, upper back, and legs.

- Stretches muscles that are often tight in the upper back.

- Counteracts forward flexion activities (such as looking down at a computer keyboard, reading, and texting on your phone).

4. Downward Facing Dog

Alternative name: Down Dog

Sanskrit name: *Adho Mukha Svanasana*

Associated chakra: Third eye (Ajna chakra), throat (Vishuddha chakra), heart (Anahata chakra), solar plexus (Manipura chakra)

Elements: Light, Ether, Air, Fire

Closely related poses: Child's Pose, Dolphin Pose

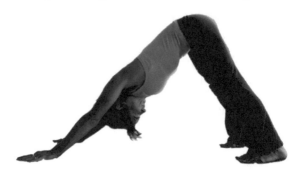

Downward Facing Dog Step-by-Step

1. You'll move from Upward Facing Dog into Downward Facing Dog on an exhale.

2. Keep your hands exactly where they are, with your fingers spread wide.

3. Tuck your toes as you simultaneously lift your hips towards the ceiling and drive your chest towards your thighs. Your body will now be in an inverted "v" position.

4. Press through your hands and straighten your legs. Your feet can stay on your tippy-toes or you can flatten your feet (heels to the floor) if you have enough flexibility in your hamstrings.

5. Create a spiral action in your arms. You do this by rolling your upper arms away from you and spiraling your forearms inwards. If you are hyper-mobile (very flexible), you should avoid locking

your elbows by keeping a micro-bend in your arms.

6. Allow your head to relax, and don't hunch your shoulders. You can nod and shake your head to make sure the base of your neck isn't tense.

Modifications

- If you have tight hamstrings, you can keep your legs slightly bent in Downward Facing Dog. It is way more important to have a straight back than straight legs! This pose is designed to lengthen the spine.

- To focus on your arm strength, you can loop an exercise band (or buckled strap) around your arms, just above the elbows. This creates tension for you to press against. You can do the same for your legs by placing an exercise band around your thighs, just above the knees. This will help you keep your legs active as you work to keep the strap taut.

Benefits

- Strengthens the entire body including the upper arms, shoulders, abdomen, and legs.

- Stretches the back of the body including the spine, calves, and hamstrings.

- Calms the mind and stimulates blood circulation: A fantastic recovery pose after a rigorous sequence that allows you to catch your breath and recenter.

- Rests the spine between strong backbends and forward bends and realigns the body.

Putting it all Together

Usually, during a Vinyasa yoga class or when performing a Sun Salutation sequence, these four poses will be incorporated with the breath, and for each inhale and exhale you will shift to a new pose. This is called "moving with the breath."

It will look and sound something like this:

"Step back into plank as you inhale, exhale down into Low Plank, inhale into Upward Facing Dog, exhale into Downward Facing Dog."

Sun Salutations

The Sun Salutations (also known as *Surya Namaskar* in Sanskrit) are a set sequence of poses that you can learn by heart and practice yourself. You don't need a yoga instructor to know what to do next—you'll know! The Sun Salutations are key fundamentals in yoga and are a wonderful place to start as a beginner.

Surya, translated from Sanskrit, means "sun" and *namaskar* means "show gratitude." In ancient Hindu traditions, the Sun Salutations were used during morning prayer as the sun rose. They've evolved over time and are now often used to warm up the body, to calm the mind, and to enter a meditative state.

The salutations are done in sync with the breath and, when repeated enough times, can be incredibly soothing for anxiety and stress. One particularly enjoyable way of doing the Sun Salutations is by completing 108 in a row. This can be exhausting for beginners, but it is tremendously calming. The number 108 is considered a sacred number in some traditions and religions (such as Buddhism, Jainism and Hinduism), and is significant in meditation (there are also 108 beads in a *mala*, for instance, which are used to count mantras while meditating).

There are a number of variations of the Sun Salutation, but the two most common are simply called A and B. We will have a close look at both.

Sun Salutation A contains fewer poses and is ideal for beginner yogis. Sun Salutation B contains a longer sequence that includes more challenging poses such as Chair Pose and Warrior I. The range of poses in both sequences are designed to open up all the areas of the body so you can work each muscle group by simply following these set series of asanas.

Sun Salutation A

1. Stand at the top of your mat with your feet hip-distance apart. You can start with your hands in Prayer Position, or with your arms by your side. This is Mountain Pose (Tadasana). Feel your feet rooting into the ground, lengthen your spine, and close your eyes if you wish. When you're ready to start, drop your hands to your side and face your palms forward (this automatically releases your shoulders back and down). Inhale and exhale here to ground yourself as you open your eyes.

2. Inhale and raise your arms above your head, gazing up at your hands and opening your heart. This pose is called upward salute (Urdhva Hastasana).

3. Exhale down to Standing Forward Fold (Uttanasana). You'll hinge from your hips, keeping a flat back, and fold forward. Your knees can be as bent as they need to be to allow your chest to rest against your legs (you can eventually progress to straight legs here).

4. Inhale as you move into Low Lunge (Anjaneyasana). You step your left foot back, and your right knee will be above your right ankle. Your hips face forward and your arms can either extend upwards to the sky as you look up, or meet at your heart center in Prayer. You may also choose to simply keep your hands towards the floor and lift your gaze.

5. Exhale to Downward Facing Dog (Adho Mukha Svanasana). You'll bring your hands back to the floor on either side of your right foot and step it back into Down Dog. Remember to focus on a straight back and bend your knees if you need. Your head stays relaxed and in line with your biceps.

6. Inhale down to Plank Pose (Phalakasana). This can be a beautiful fluid movement. If your Downward Facing Dog was positioned correctly, your hands and feet will stay exactly where they are on the mat, while you simply roll forward into plank. Remember to keep your shoulders directly above your wrists and engage your core and glutes.

7. Exhale to Low Plank (Chaturanga Dandasana). Your elbows hug your ribcage, and your core is engaged.

8. Inhale to Upward Facing Dog (Urdhva Mukha Svanasana). Lift your heart center and push up to

straight arms, shoulders over the wrists, thighs and knees lifted off the mat. Keep your spine long and your core tight.

9. Exhale to Downward Facing Dog.

10. Inhale to low lunge on the same side so your right foot steps forward. Bring your hands to your mat (if they aren't there already) on either side of your right foot.

11. Exhale to Standing Forward Fold, bringing your left foot forward to meet your right at the top of your mat.

12. Inhale to upward salute, raising your arms to the sky and gazing upward.

13. Exhale, bringing your hands to Prayer at your heart center, or next to your sides, returning to Mountain Pose.

14. Repeat this on the left side to complete one full round of Sun Salutation A.

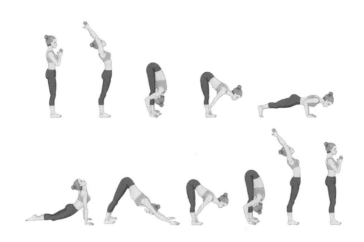

Sun Salutation B

1. Start at the top of your mat in Mountain Pose.
    Take a few moments to ground yourself and find
    your center.

2. Inhale and bend your knees deeply as you sweep
    your hands up and come into Chair Pose
    (Utkatasana). Your upper arms will brush past
    your ears. Try to keep your knees in line and don't
    allow them to overshoot your toes–your spine
    needs to stay long. Keep your gaze fixed on a
    point directly in front of you. We'll go into much
    more detail on Chair Pose later on in this chapter,
    so don't worry if you're not sure how to do it just
    yet.

3. Exhale into Standing Forward Fold by straightening your legs and bringing your hands to the mat on either side of your feet or as low on your legs as you can reach.

4. Inhale to "halfway lift"—Half Standing Forward Fold (Ardha Uttanasana)—where you look forward and straighten your back, lifting onto your fingertips in front of your feet (or alternatively resting your palms on your shins).

5. Exhale to Low Plank (Chaturanga Dandasana). You do this by bending your knees deeply and pressing your palms firmly into the mat. Gaze in front of your toes as you exhale, engaging your abdominals to support your spine. You can either jump back or step back into Low Plank. You'll land (or end up) with your elbows bent, and shoulders in line with your elbows.

6. Inhale to Upward Facing Dog. Roll over your toes and press your chest between your upper arms, gazing forward or slightly upward. Remember to keep your knees and thighs off of the floor with the tops of your feet firmly on your mat.

7. Exhale to Downward Facing Dog. Remember to keep your spine long and your shoulders and neck relaxed.

8. Inhale to Warrior I (Virabhadrasana I). You do this by raising your right leg while in Downward Facing Dog and stepping the right foot between your hands. Your right knee is bent, and your right foot is facing forwards. Turn your left toes slightly out, and make sure your feet are hip-width apart. Raise your arms to the sky as you press into the outer edge of your left foot. Your weight should be spread evenly with your hips facing forward. You can keep your arms straight or join your palms together as you gaze upward.

9. Exhale to Low Plank (Chaturanga) by bringing your hands on either side of your right foot and stepping back as you lower body down.

10. Inhale to Upward Facing Dog.

11. Exhale to Downward Facing Dog.

12. Inhale to Warrior I on the left side. From Downward Facing Dog, step forward with your left foot into Warrior I. Your right foot will be turned slightly out, your left foot facing forward, and left knee bent. Raise your arms to the sky and gaze upward.

13. Exhale to Low Plank.

14. Inhale to Upward Facing Dog.

15. Exhale to Downward Facing Dog. You can stay here for a few breaths as you recenter and realign.

16. Bend your knees deeply and gaze forward at your hands. Come onto the balls of your feet and hop, float, or step to the top of your mat.

17. Inhale as you lift your gaze and extend your spine into Halfway Lift.

18. Exhale into Standing Forward Fold.

19. Inhale into Chair Pose, lifting your arms above your head.

20. Exhale and press your feet into the ground as you straighten your legs, bringing your palms together at your heart center. Stand here in Mountain Pose with your eyes closed for a few rounds of breath before repeating the entire sequence as many times as you desire.

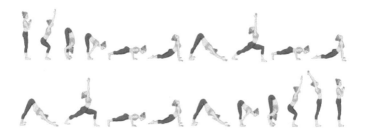

More Foundational Poses

You'll find that after doing a few rounds of sun salutations, you'll actually know quite a few key yoga poses and transitions. I'll now guide you through some other common asanas you're likely to come across during a yoga class. Here are the 15 additional poses we'll cover in this chapter:

- Cat/Cow Pose
- Child's Pose
- Crescent Moon Pose
- Warrior I, II, and III
- Reverse Warrior
- Extended Side Angle
- Chair Pose
- Triangle Pose
- Dancer's Pose
- Tree Pose
- Seated Forward Fold
- Cobra Pose
- Bridge Pose
- Shoulder Stand
- Corpse Pose

Cat/Cow Pose

Sanskrit name: *Marjaryasana Bitilasana*

This is a beautiful centering and realigning movement that is often performed near the beginning of a yoga class or sequence. It warms up your back muscles and is a great place to start implementing the ocean breath (we'll cover how to perform this regulating breath in a different chapter).

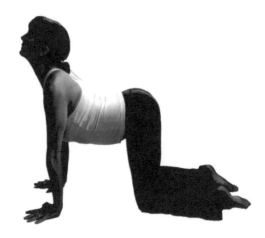

1. Start in Tabletop Position with your wrists directly beneath your shoulders and your knees below your hips. Your back should be straight and your core engaged.

2. Relax your neck in this neutral position and make sure your fingers are facing forwards and are spread wide apart. Concentrate on "pushing the ground away."

3. Inhale into Cow Pose. Your back arches and your belly leans toward the mat. Gaze straight ahead or slightly upward. Focus on opening your collar bones and expanding your chest.

4. Exhale into Cat Pose. Round your upper, middle, and lower back, and tuck your chin towards your chest. Imagine yourself as a cat getting a good stretch in the morning.

5. Inhale to Cow Pose, exhale to Cat Pose. Repeat as many times as you wish. A good rule of thumb is about five rounds.

Modifications

If your knees get sore from kneeling too long, you can place them on a blanket or rolled up mat. You may initially struggle with your balance, so it can help to space your knees and hands slightly wider, or tuck your toes under for more support.

Be careful that you don't over-compress your spine in Cow Pose, and don't allow your hips to push back when you arch into Cat Pose.

Benefits

The movement of Cat/Cow Pose creates space and mobility in the spine and opens the front and back of the body. This simple alternation of positions strengthens your back, core, and neck. It also releases tension in the lower back and helps to align and stretch stiff muscles.

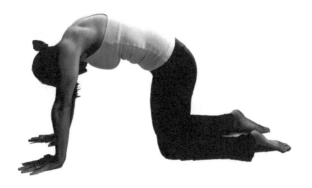

Child's Pose

Sanskrit name: *Balasana*

This is a foundational resting pose that you can return to at any time in your practice. If you feel you need to slow down or that your body is taking strain, then Child's Pose is your go-to asana.

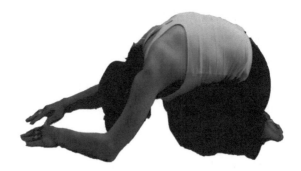

1. Sit on your knees and widen them to the sides of your mat (this creates more space in your hips). You can also keep your knees together to create more length through your spine. Discern what your body needs most today.

2. Bring your big toes to touch and sit back on your heels.

3. Lay your chest onto or between your thighs. You should feel your hips settle.

4. Reach your arms forward to extend your spine and place your forehead on the mat. Try to extend your fingers as far as possible.

5. You can also do a slight variation of Child's Pose (called Embryo Pose) where you rest your arms at your sides (hands touching your heels and palms up). This opens up your shoulder blades more, but you'll feel less of a stretch in your back.

Modifications

Remember that lengthening your spine is the goal, not getting your hips onto your heels. You can even place a blanket or block between the backs of your thighs and calves if this is more comfortable. Alternatively, you can place a bolster or block between your legs if this feels more supportive.

Your forehead may not be able to reach the floor, and in this case, you can rest on a block instead. This will keep the shape and proper alignment of the pose without overextending.

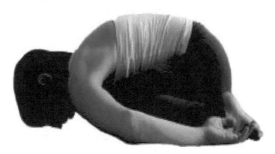

Benefits

Child's Pose is fantastic for a gentle opening of the hips while lengthening the spine. It slows your heart rate and calms the mind. It also helps to reduce stress and fatigue and is a wonderful posture to realign your body after twisted poses.

Crescent Moon Pose

Sansrkit name: *Anjaneyasana*

Crescent Moon Pose is also called Low Lunge. It's a stunning transitional pose.

1. From Downward Facing Dog, exhale and step your right foot between your hands at the front of your mat. Place your left knee on the floor and as you inhale, raise your arms above your head. You can keep them parallel or bring your palms to touch.

2. Your shoulders should be stacked above your hips.

3. Lengthen your torso and extend your spine.

4. Your front knee should be above the ankle (not past).

5. Hug your front heel in toward the middle of your mat without moving its position.

6. Your back toes can be untucked with balanced pressure against all your toe nails, or tucked under with your heel pressed back.

7. Your front hip moves back, and your back hip moves forward.

8. Engage the glutes of your back leg.

9. Gaze up at your hands and keep the back of your neck long.

10. Repeat on the other side.

Modifications

You can keep your front knee behind your ankle if needed.

If your back knee needs extra support, you can place it on a rolled up towel. Don't put too much weight on this back leg—rather, lunge deeper with your front leg.

You can rest your hands on your front thigh if you feel off balance with your arms raised.

Gaze forward instead of upward if you need more stability.

Benefits

Crescent Moon Pose strengthens your quadriceps and glutes. This improves the stamina and endurance of your upper legs. The pose also opens your psoas muscle and hips, expands your chest, and opens your shoulders.

Crescent Moon Pose also relieves sciatica pain and lengthens your spine. It also improves your balance, coordination, and core stability.

Warrior I

Sanskrit name: *Virabhadrasana A*

This pose requires strength and balance, but is brilliant for focus and self-awareness.

1. You'll likely come into this asana from Downward Facing Dog. Step one foot forward between your hands with your front knee stacked above the ankle. Eventually, you want to aim to have your front thigh parallel to the ground.

2. Ground your back foot at a 45-degree angle, keeping the outer blade of the back foot grounded and active.

3. Straighten your back leg, keeping it strong and engaged by contracting your thigh muscle and "pulling up your kneecap". Your feet should be approximately hip-width apart.

4. Square your hips and shoulders forward. Your hips should be aligned, which usually requires you to focus on shifting the front hip slightly back, and the hip of the back leg slightly forward.

5. Your shoulders are stacked above your hips, and your spine is long.

6. Inhale and raise your hands above your head and, if you're able to find your balance, glance up at your hands. You can keep your arms shoulder-width apart, or you can bring your palms together.

Make sure that you don't scrunch your shoulders up. Concentrate on pulling them down and away from your ears.

Modifications

If you struggle with your balance, or if there is too much strain on your front leg, you can shorten your stance to make it easier. You can also bend your front knee less.

Keeping your arms parallel is less challenging than joining the palms above your head. You may also find it helps to place your hands on your hips instead for extra support.

Instead of gazing upward, you can gaze forward to help with keeping your balance.

Benefits

Warrior I increases the flexibility and strength of your hips, and sculpts your thighs, calves, shoulders, arms, and back. The pose opens your chest and upper back, elongates your spine and abdomen, and stretches the psoas muscle (a common area of tension).

Warrior II

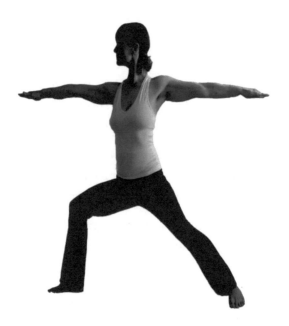

Sanskrit name: *Virabhadrasana B*

This powerful pose lives up to its name. It's one you're bound to feel strong in and is a great pose to focus on building endurance, clearing your mind, and letting go of all distractions.

1. You will usually enter this pose from Warrior I or a Low Lunge.

2. Your front knee is bent and your front thigh should be parallel to the ground.

3. Your back leg is extended with your back heel grounded (press the outer edge of your foot into

the ground), and toes turned in to face the side of your mat.

4. To make sure your feet are in the correct alignment, imagine a straight line drawn from the heel of your front foot to the middle of the arch of your back foot.

5. Your hips are squared with the side of your mat, equal, and aligned (the incorrect tendency is to bring the back hip forward).

6. Your upper body should be completely straight, so keep your shoulders stacked directly above your hips.

7. Extend your arms out to the sides to form a T-shape. You can gaze over your front fingers (the direction your bent front leg is facing).

8. Relax your shoulders, and remember to breathe!

Modifications

If Warrior II is too intense for your front thigh muscles, then you can shorten your stance. This will allow your thigh to be higher than parallel to the ground, which makes it less intense.

Your front knee can also be behind your ankle instead of right above it. This also makes the pose easier. Remember to never go the opposite way, however. You don't want your knee to go past your ankles and towards your toes–this can damage your knee.

If you find that you battle to balance in this pose, you can gaze straight ahead (the way your hips are facing) instead of over your fingers.

Benefits

Warrior II strengthens your legs, ankles, hips, and arms. It opens your hips, chest, and lungs. It's also a wonderful pose for toning and sculpting your glutes and thighs, improving blood circulation, building stamina and concentration, and developing balance and stability.

Warrior III

Sanskrit name: *Virabhadrasana C* or *Digasana*

This is a strong balancing posture that takes focus and quite a bit of wobblies in the beginning. However, once you get it right, you'll feel a tremendous sense of accomplishment!

1. It's easy to start this pose from Warrior I.

2. Keep your arms raised above your head, straighten your front leg, and lean forward. Your body should tip to reach a 90-degree angle, with your back leg stretched out behind you, parallel to the ground. Your body will form one straight, parallel line, from the tips of your toes of your raised leg to the tips of your fingers.

3. You can keep your arms parallel or bring your palms to touch. Your head should be relaxed and your gaze at a point on the mat in front of you.

4. Engage your standing leg by contracting your quadriceps.

5. To improve your grounding and balance, it helps to spread your weight evenly on your standing foot and spread your toes wide.

Modifications

There is a variation to Warrior III that is often used in popular classes. The pose is called Airplane Pose and involves the same position, but instead of extending your arms forward in front of you, you reach your arms back along your sides like wings. Keep your hands active and extended toward the wall behind you.

If your hamstrings aren't strong enough to hold this pose with a straight leg, you can bend your standing leg as much as you need.

Instead of extending your hands in front of you, you can bring them together at your heart center, or alternatively, rest them on your standing thigh for additional support.

While you're learning to find your balance, you can also press your lifted foot against a wall for stability.

Be careful that you don't dip your chest below your hips and don't tense your neck or jaw.

Benefits

Warrior III strengthens your legs, glutes, and back muscles. It's also an excellent workout for your triceps, biceps, and abs. You'll naturally develop your balance and concentration while getting your blood flowing!

Reverse Warrior

Sanskrit name: *Viparita Virabhadrasana B*

Reverse Warrior is a pose that often follows Warrior II and then leads into Extended Side Angle.

1. From Warrior II, while keeping your legs in exactly the same position, inhale and turn the palm of your front hand to face the sky.

2. Reach your front arm up and along the top ear. You want to try and create a spiral in your top upper arm by aiming your pinky finger towards the floor.

3. The idea is to lengthen the side of your body. Think about lifting and lengthening your torso, as opposed to reaching backward.

4. Your back hand should rest gently on your back thigh or calf, depending on your flexibility. There should be little to no weight in this back hand.

5. Keep your front leg bent the entire time, with your front knee stacked above the ankle.

6. Your back leg provides the strength and stability to hold the posture, so make sure it is engaged.

7. Gaze up toward your extended arm.

Modifications

As with all the Warrior poses, you can shorten your stance to make the asana less challenging. Once again, you can have less bend in your front knee for additional stability.

Remember this is a side stretch, not a backbend—so you shouldn't be feeling tension in your back at all. It helps to imagine your back is against a wall to prevent you leaning backwards or forwards in the pose.

Benefits

Reverse Warrior is wonderful for lengthening the side of your body and creates space in your ribcage. It strengthens your legs and glutes and is a fantastic hip-opener.

Extended Side Angle

Sanskrit name: *Utthita Parsvakonasana*

Extended Side Angle is commonly a transition pose. You'll often do this straight after Warrior II or reverse warrior, and then usually from Extended Side Angle into a low lunge.

1. Position your arms and feet in a Warrior II stance.

2. Rest your front arm on the thigh of your front knee (this will be as close to parallel to the ground as you can manage).

3. Reach your back arm alongside your ear, without placing any weight on your front arm. Be careful that you don't lean forward. Keep your shoulders and torso in the same plane as your hips.

4. Wrap your top shoulder and orient your pinky finger toward the floor. This creates a spiral in your upper arm.

5. Keep the outer blade of your back foot grounded for stability.

6. Rotate the top side of your ribcage towards the sky. This is a chest-opening pose.

7. Gaze towards the sky and your top hand.

Modifications

Advanced versions of this pose include the Extended Side Angle Bind. This is where your bottom arm loops around your front leg, your top arm reaches behind you, and you clasp your hands to form a bind.

Another variation is to place the bottom hand on the floor next to the front foot to extend the stretch.

Beginners can gaze forward or down instead of upward. It's also absolutely fine to place your front hand on a block or to shorten your stance and decrease the angle of the bend in your front knee.

Benefits

Extended Side Angle strengthens your hips, knees, and thighs. It opens the entire body, including the back, abdomen, chest, and shoulders. This pose stimulates and massages your internal organs which improves digestion and also increases your stamina, balance, and coordination.

Chair Pose

Sanskrit name: *Utkatasana*

Chair Pose is one that most of us love and hate at the same time. It builds heat, strengthens your muscles, enhances focus, and provides a great sense of achievement. However, after a few seconds, it becomes incredibly challenging.

1. From a standing position, such as Mountain Pose, bend your knees and imagine you're sitting in a chair. Shift your weight to your heels and reach your arms above your head (alongside your ears).

2. Make sure your knees are in line with each other and that they aren't extending past your toes. Speaking of toes, your big toes should be touching in a traditional Chair Pose. However, if you need more stability, you can set your feet at hip-distance apart.

3. Lift your chest up and forward.

4. Your arms can also come to Prayer at your heart center (*anjali mudra*) or on your hips if you need the support and balance.

5. Gaze at a single point in front of you and breathe.

6. The deeper you sink (or "sit"), the more challenging the pose becomes. Eventually, the goal will be to get your thighs parallel to the ground.

7. Keep your back straight and long throughout.

Modifications

Straighten your knees to a more comfortable position if you're struggling to sit low.

If your lower back is hurting, or if you're pregnant, keep your feet hip-distance apart.

Benefits

Chair Pose is an incredibly strong posture. It sculpts your quads and glutes, and tones your entire back. This pose increases your heart rate and improves blood circulation, stimulates your metabolism, and generates heat.

Triangle Pose

Sanskrit name: *Trikonasana*

Triangle Pose is one that we often see on Instagram. It's beautiful to look at because of its symmetry and form. Although it can be challenging to master your alignment in this pose, it's certainly a feel-good one. You'll feel both sides of your waist stretch, and your body will likely enjoy the sensation of the straight lines.

1. Start with your legs and arms in a Warrior II position. Straighten your front leg and engage both your legs by contracting your thigh muscles and glutes.

2. Ground into the outer blade of your back foot. This creates a slight internal rotation of your back thigh.

3. Reach as far forward as you can with your front arm, as if you're reaching for a glass on a shelf. Keep your feet firmly rooted and don't move your legs. You should feel a lengthening on both sides of your torso.

4. Turn your palms to face the same direction as your hips and then tilt your torso down. Your bottom hand will either rest against your calf, on your shin, or on a block. Stretch your top arm to the sky, keeping it directly in line with your bottom arm. Your arms should form a straight line from fingertip to fingertip. Make sure there is no weight on your bottom hand.

5. Now, gaze up at your top fingers.

Modifications

You can place your hand higher up your front leg if you're struggling to balance (just don't place it directly on your knee).

Instead of gazing up at your top hand, you can gaze forward or down. This helps with stability in the beginning.

Shorten your stance for more support, and bend the front knee slightly if your hamstrings are tight.

Benefits

Triangle Pose strengthens the thighs, knees, hips, and ankles. It opens the hips and chest and stimulates the internal organs, which improves digestion. The pose is a great one for creating space in the upper back and muscles along the spine.

Dancer's Pose

Sanskrit name: *Natarajasana*

This is one of the most graceful and beautiful yoga poses. There is an advanced version where both hands extend past your head and grab your foot from above (this can be achieved by using a strap at first). Let's start with the basic Dancer's Pose.

1. From Mountain Pose, bend your knees and ground your weight onto one foot.

2. Place the ball of your other foot on the floor in preparation. Try to get to just resting on your big toe.

3. Engage the thigh of your standing leg and lift your kneecap up.

4. Lift the opposite leg up and back while bending the knee.

5. Hold the inside of your raised foot with the hand of the same side. Reach your other arm upward and forwards.

6. Start with both knees together and get your balance while gazing straight ahead.

7. Now, kick back with your raised foot in the air while lifting your chest. Make sure your standing leg is straight.

8. Create this standing backbend by increasing the tension between your upper body and back leg. Kick your foot back against your hand while leaning forward.

9. Your chest should always be higher than your hips.

10. Keep your hips in line with each other.

11. Gaze forward and upward.

Modifications

You can bend your standing leg and use a strap on your lifted foot. Be careful to not let your raised leg's hip flare open.

You also don't need to lift your leg all the way up. Even if you just stand with your foot in your hand and both knees together, that is totally fine. Move at your own pace.

Benefits

Dancer's Pose opens your chest, shoulders, upper back, lower back, hips, thighs, and abdomen. It strengthens and sculpts your thighs and lengthens your spine. This posture also improves focus, balance, posture, and flexibility.

Tree Pose

Sanskrit name: *Vrksasana*

Tree Pose is a powerful balancing posture that helps improve concentration and grounds your body and emotions. It's a brilliant way for beginners to practice balancing and standing on one leg.

1. Start in Mountain Pose with your hands at your sides.

2. Shift your weight to your right foot and raise your left leg up, placing the sole of your left foot on the inner thigh of your right leg. If you can't get it

that high, you can also place it on your right calf (but avoid the knee).

3. Root through your standing leg and spread your toes wide as you find your balance. Engage this standing leg by activating your thigh muscle.

4. Lengthen your spine and lift your chest, gazing at one steady point in front of you.

5. Relax your shoulders (don't hunch them up to your ears) and place your palms together in Prayer. You can also raise your arms to the sky if you prefer, leaving them parallel or with palms joined above your head.

6. The more firmly your sole is pushed against your thigh, the stronger your balance will be.

7. Your hips should be aligned parallel to the floor (you may need to drop the hip of your raised leg to come in line with the standing hip).

8. Focus on bringing your raised knee in line with your hips. In other words, not leaning too far forwards.

9. Stay here for a few, focused breaths before switching to the opposite side.

Modifications

If you keep losing your balance, even with your foot on your calf, you can place the tip of your big toe on your mat for more support. It also helps you feel less wobbly if you put your hands on your hips.

Advanced yogis can place their raised leg in Half Lotus Position, where your foot will rest in the crease of your standing hip. This can also eventually become a bind (your opposite hand reaches behind your back and grabs the toes of your lotus foot).

Benefits

Tree pose improves your focus, posture, and balance. It also increases the flexibility of your hip joints and knees, while strengthening the thighs and calves. Your feet are stronger, you feel more grounded, and it builds confidence. Tree Pose is fantastic for opening the hips and inner thighs and tightening your core.

Seated Forward Fold

Sanskrit name: *Paschimottanasana*

The most important thing to remember with this lengthening posture is that the focus should be on elongating your spine and not on straightening your legs or getting your head to your shins.

1. Sit down on your mat and extend your legs straight out in front of you. Your feet should be touching and active (feet flexed).

2. Ground your sitting bones (your pelvic floor) by pressing them into the mat.

3. Inhale and reach your arms above your head, lengthening your spine as much as you can.

4. Exhale and reach forward, folding over your thighs. Your aim is to get your chest onto your thighs, without hunching your back. So bend forward from your hips and reach your chest over your thighs. Bend your knees as much as you need to in order to achieve this. As you get more flexible in your hamstrings, your legs will stretch straighter and straighter.

5. Your hands can hold your feet, ankles, or shins. Your head should be relaxed.

6. When you're at the peak of this pose, your forehead will be on your shins, your chest on your thighs, your legs completely straight, and your hands around your feet.

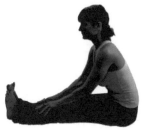 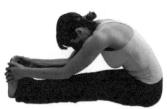

Modifications

Remember to bend your knees as much as you need, though you still want to feel a stretch in your hamstrings.

Focus on lengthening your back. Don't be afraid to push yourself a little in this one!

You can also place support under your knees, such as a bolster or rolled-up blanket. If your back gets sore, you can sit on a block or bolster to decrease the angle of your hip bend.

Just be sure that you don't hunch your shoulders or collapse your chest. Keep your spine long and straight.

Benefits

The Seated Forward Fold opens and stretches the entire back and lengthens the hamstrings and calves. The more you do this pose, the more flexible your hamstrings will become (this is especially exciting if you're doing all you can to touch your toes when you're standing up!).

The pose also calms your mind and central nervous system and is a great stress reliever.

Cobra Pose

Sanskrit name: *Bhujangasana*

Cobra Pose is a heart-opening asana that looks easier than it is. It is a backbend that strengthens your lower spine and engages your entire body.

1. Start by lying on your belly with your forehead on your mat. Your legs should be together and your toes untucked (tops of the feet pressing into the mat).

2. Place your palms face-down on your mat, directly below your shoulders.

3. Squeeze your legs together from the tops of your thighs to your ankles. Keep this engagement throughout the pose. It helps to lift your knees slightly as this immediately activates your thigh muscles. You can also imagine rotating your inner thighs towards the ceiling.

4. Hug your elbows towards your body and slide your shoulders down. In other words, pull them down and away from your ears.

5. Inhale and gently lift your chest off the floor. You don't want any weight in your hands. In fact, if you can hover your hands slightly above your mat, that is ideal. You want to use the strength of your core and lower back to lift your chest, not your arms. Your chest will move forward and up.

6. Keep your gaze straight ahead or slightly upward—but don't crane your neck. You want your neck to be long and your chin slightly tucked.

7. Push your hips into the mat and engage your glutes.

8. Exhale and lower your chest back down to your mat, followed by your forehead.

Modifications

You can place a block between your thighs to support your lower back. You only need to lift your upper body a little off the floor.

You can use your hands for support in the beginning.

Remember to keep your legs active, your feet engaged (don't splay them to the sides), and don't hunch your shoulders. If you feel a tweak in your lower back at any point then you are going too far for your body's current capability.

Benefits

Cobra Pose increases your spinal strength and flexibility and opens your chest, lungs, shoulders, and heart. It also strengthens your upper body and massages your internal organs which improves digestion. This pose also helps relieve stress and fatigue and improves blood circulation, especially in the pelvic area.

Bridge Pose

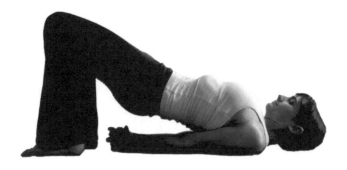

Sanskrit name: *Setu Bandha Sarvangasana*

Bridge Pose is a wonderful asana to counteract a lot of core and abdominal work. It's usually performed towards the end of class as you're cooling down.

1. Lie flat on your back with your arms by your sides and palms facing down. Bend your knees, bringing your feet flat on the floor. Your feet should be hip-distance apart with your toes pointing forward.

2. Place your feet close to your hips. You should be able to graze your heels with your fingers. Your knees must be directly above your ankles.

3. Press your hands and feet into the floor and lift your hips as high as you can.

4. Shimmy your shoulders underneath your body and create a shelf with your upper back as support.

5. If you have the flexibility you can interlace your hands underneath your hips on the mat.

6. Your arms should be straight and your feet active.

7. Lift your chest towards your chin, but keep your neck relaxed.

8. Hold the pose as long as you're comfortable to do so.

Modifications

You can place a block between your thighs for extra stability and to ensure proper alignment.

If you have lower back pain you can also place a block under your sacrum for additional support.

While you're gaining strength it's absolutely fine to only raise your hips slightly off the ground.

Benefits

Bridge Pose opens your chest and spine, and lengthens your abdominal wall. It stimulates your abdominal organs, lungs, and thyroid. Your lung capacity increases, your thighs and glutes tone, your digestion improves, and your lower back strengthens.

Shoulder Stand

Sanskrit name: *Salamba Sarvangasana*

Shoulder Stand is a stimulating yet restorative pose. It's usually done towards the end of class and is held for at least five breaths.

1. Lie down on your mat and bend your knees with your feet flat on the floor.

2. Lift your hips up, similar to how you would in Bridge Pose. Place your hands on your mid to lower back, with fingers facing your buttocks.

3. Gently push yourself up, lifting both legs to the sky. Your fingers will now be pointing towards the ceiling. Your elbows need to be tight against your body.

4. Your shoulders, hips, and heels should all be in one straight line.

5. Keep your big toes together with a small space between your heels.

6. Keep your feet active, as if you're standing with flat feet against the ceiling.

Modifications

You can place a folded blanket under your shoulders and upper back for extra support and to increase the angle of your neck and head (the constriction on your throat will be less).

You can also modify this pose by lying with your hips and back flat on the floor, but still raising your legs to the sky (this variation is called Legs Up The Wall pose).

Don't move your head from side to side in this pose. Gaze up at your feet the entire time.

Benefits

Shoulder Stand soothes your brain and central nervous system. It also stimulates your thyroid gland and lymph system. This pose massages your abdominal organs and opens your shoulders. It's an amazing pose to relieve fatigue and insomnia.

Corpse Pose

Sanskrit name: *Savasana*

Ahh, the end of class! Corpse Pose, also known as Rest Pose, is where we can relax and release, possibly do a meditation or visualization, and just absorb all the benefits of our practice. There is no right or wrong way to do this one. The main thing is that you're comfortable, relaxed, and allowing every part of your body to let go.

1. Lie flat on your back and extend your legs out. Allow your feet to relax and flop to the side.

2. Your arms can be about 45 degrees away from the body, with palms facing the sky. This is a receptive, open gesture.

3. Move your head from side to side to make sure it is relaxed and that you're not tensing your neck.

4. Close your eyes and exhale deeply.

5. Relax and breathe naturally.

Modifications

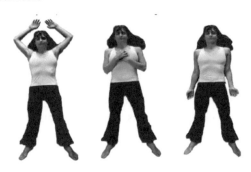

You can have a support under your head, neck, or knees if it makes this pose more comfortable for you. You can also place an eye cushion over your eyes. This creates complete darkness and is incredibly calming.

Benefits

Corpse Pose is deeply relaxing, takes no effort, and deepens your natural breath. It allows your body to absorb and integrate all you did during your yoga practice, and creates a quiet, healing space for your body and mind.

Chapter 6:

Lock It

There are some yoga practices that can seem strange at first. Usually, yoga is all about opening the body so that energy can flow freely, fully expanding and releasing our breath, and calming down our nervous system.

However, some practices intensify the flow of energy and then restrict it, elevate the heart rate, and involve holding the breath for extended periods of time. The internal yogic locks, also known as *bandhas*, are examples of techniques that seem to aim for these paradoxical effects.

In this chapter, we'll discover why it's sometimes necessary to close off the throat (*Jalandhara bandha*), or what the contraction and lifting of the abdomen (*Uddiyana bandha*) achieves, and how drawing inward at the center of the pelvic floor (*Mula bandha*) can have multiple benefits.

At first, it can look and feel strange. Uddiyana bandha, for example, sucks the stomach in so much that the ribs protrude and the abdomen becomes hollow. In Mula bandha, we're told to imagine we're preventing ourselves from urinating, and the Jalandhara bandha can feel rather claustrophobic as we cut off our air supply. It may sound bizarre, and yet these practices make perfect sense once you come to terms with their context.

It's important to know why the bandhas are practiced to fully understand the intelligence behind them. We'll delve into the reasoning by looking at theories drawn from Hatha, Tantra, and Kundalini Yoga.

Let's start at the beginning.

Energy Patterns in the Body

Our bodies are filled with energy at so many different levels. There are patterns of energy circulating in our cells, and millions of long lines of energy coursing through our veins and even pulsating through our subtle, emotional bodies.

There are a number of complex interactions going on in our bodies at any given moment and as long as we are alive, the different parts of our body are active and engaged.

According to yogic philosophy (Sovik, 2015), all the energy in our bodies is a configuration of five primary energy functions (vayus), or five forces of *Prana* (upper-case P). The two most prominent are *prana* (lower-case p) and *apana*.

Before we go any further, allow me to explain the difference between Prana and *prana*.

Prana (upper-case P) is a Sanskrit term that means "life force." It's the energy within and around our physical bodies. Some other Eastern philosophies refer to this as "Chi" (sometimes spelled "Qi"), and in the Western world, it is sometimes thought of as our spirit. It's the part of us that continues after our physical body dies.

Many believe that Prana is carried and transmitted through the breath (prana with a lower-case p). This flow of energy via our breath is connected to our spine. Various yogic philosophies believe that as we inhale the pranic energy flows up our spine, and then flows down our spine as we exhale. This energy pathway is often referred to as *nadis*.

Prana itself is divided into different categories, which are essentially different forms of life force. These five categories are prana, apana, samana, vyana, and udana.

As we said earlier, the two most prominent are prana and apana. These are the forces that regulate how we receive and eliminate energy. The acquisition of energy (where it originally comes from) is prana (or breath), and is characterized by an upward-moving process or filling up. This is connected to the chest and throat. Of course, the significance here makes sense, because these are the organs we use when we breathe in air, drink water, and eat food (all sources of energy).

Apana is an emptying out energy or downward-moving process. It's connected to the lower abdomen and pelvic floor. This energy governs urination, defecation, and the menstrual cycle.

The third component of Prana is called samana. This is centered at the navel region and governs the absorption of energy through digestion and the generation of internal heat. This is also where the solar plexus chakra is located. It's a hub of fiery power that distributes energy to the rest of our bodies (it does this through channels and pathways also known as nadis—you may remember that from earlier on).

The fourth component of Prana is known as vyana, which exists throughout the body and is responsible for circulation and expansiveness. It moves in a circular and pulsating manner and is connected very closely to the cardiac system.

The fifth and final component is udana. This is located in the throat area and governs speech and expression. It's an upward-moving energy that depends on the correct functioning of the other vayus.

The activities of these five Pranic energies comprise one layer or dimension in the pattern of human energy.

To fully understand how yogic locks work, we need to go even further down the rabbit hole and take a look at two additional dimensions of energy.

Dimension One: The Merging of Energies and Sushumna

Our energy shifts as we go through our day. The life force (Prana) that moves within us is rooted in our bodies with two internal energies. They can also be seen as modes of functioning. The two energies work together and, depending on the flow and merging of these, our overall experience is affected.

The first of these two internal energies is often described as a solar, masculine, rational, active, heating form of energy. In Chinese philosophy, it is known as yang, and in Sanskrit it is expressed by the syllable "ha."

This masculine energy flows in a channel (nadi) known as *pingala*. This line of energy ends in the right nostril. I promise this will all make sense soon, so stay with me!

The second internal energy is described by words such as lunar, feminine, intuitive, receptive, and cooling. It's symbolized by the Chinese yin, and is expressed in Sanskrit with the syllable "tha." It flows through a nadi known as *ida* which ends in the left nostril.

These two energies wrap around each other and oscillate through the day in our bodies. They shape our experiences and influence our physical and mental functioning.

Interestingly, when these two Sanskrit syllables are joined (*ha* and *tha*) they form the word *hatha*. This is a system of yoga that is designed to regulate human self-awareness, primarily through the breath and by transforming the flow of energy.

Kundalini yoga practitioners describe how these two energies of life integrate with each other and how they can merge into one central stream of energy. When they work in harmony like this, there is a transcendental awareness and ripening of the mind. This happens through the Prana flowing upward in a single, central channel along our spinal column. This channel is called *sushumna* and is sometimes illustrated or depicted as a serpent coiled around the spine. In traditional Indian culture, it is believed that this merging of two separate, yet complementary energies, leads to liberation.

Dimension Two: The Spinal Axis Poles

The second influence on the fluctuations of our internal energy arises from the polarity of our spinal axis. The top part of the spine is the positive or northern pole, and the lower part is the negative or southern pole.

When our thoughts and actions are driven by instinct, with very little self-reflection or inner awareness, then the patterns of energy are driven primarily by the lower energy centers of our spinal axis. This is where our primal, animal instinct resides. You'll have experienced this when you had a "gut feeling" about something or reacted from impulse instead of rational thought. It's often a flight or fight sensation, and the mind becomes dominated by fears, cravings, and desires. There's a strong urge to be in control.

However, as self-awareness grows (such as through meditation or other yoga practices), these base energies can be transformed. Fear can evolve to fearlessness and cravings can yield to moderation.

The Three Internal Locks

Now that you have a foundational understanding of the energy system in our bodies, the three yogic locks will probably make more sense. They are designed to bring order to these complex energetic interactions, with the ultimate goal of using the body as a tool to develop self-awareness.

These three locks were first developed by tantric masters and later adapted in the Hatha yoga tradition (Sovik, 2015). The Throat Lock, Stomach Lock, and Root Lock are fundamental yogic practices. You can learn them fairly easily and refine them over time.

We'll go into much more detail in just a bit, but I would like to give you a quick overview first so that you have a firm understanding of where this is all going.

The Throat and Root Locks are made to seal the upper and lower end of the spinal column (the two poles).

It is believed that the Throat Lock temporarily stops prana from moving upward, which restricts the flow of energy through the ida and pingala channels. You may remember that fiery masculine energy flows through pingala, ending in the right nostril, and cooling feminine energy flows through ida, ending in the left nostril. The Throat Lock restricts the flow through both these nadis.

The Root Lock blocks the downward movement of apana (that "emptying out" energy that we spoke about) and pulls this energy from the base of our spine back toward the navel region.

When these upward and downward energies are restricted, they are forced to merge together in the center of our bodies. They rub against one another to generate heat and produce a tremendous amount of combined, concentrated energy. This heat is magnified by applying the Stomach Lock at the same time.

The force of this restricted and highly concentrated energy increases with practice, and depends on how long the locks are held and if they are done in isolation or together. It is said that advanced practitioners are able to create intense heat and this, combined with breath retention, awakens their awareness. This powerful merging of energy then travels upward along the center of the spine up the sushumna nadi or channel (you may recall the image of the serpent coiling around the spine). This energy moves from the base of the spine toward the apex, and our energy shifts from fear and instinct-driven cravings to illuminated self-awareness or transcendence. Ultimately, this is the goal of yoga as a whole: Liberation.

Learning how to Perform the Locks

It's important to remember that by simply manipulating some muscles and performing subtle movements, you aren't going to miraculously change your deep-rooted patterns of thinking overnight. Not only do the locks take time to learn and master, but they also need to be practiced along with other yoga disciplines such as meditation, yoga asanas, and breathwork. Even then, it can take years of dedication to achieve dramatic results. However, you will immediately notice some physical and mental benefits, which will improve as your yoga practice deepens. Your main goal should be to foster internal awareness and learn to sense the subtle changes of energy in your body when you perform the locks.

The physical and mental benefits you may start to notice after regular practice include:

- Improving digestion and elimination.
- Increasing energy throughout your day.
- Cleansing of energy channels (feeling more grounded and less stressed).
- Toning the visceral organs.
- Preparing the mind for meditation.
- Improving concentration.
- Relieving depression and anxiety.

As these three yogic locks are extremely stimulating and involve a high concentration of energy in one area, you need to take some precautions. It's advised that you don't attempt them if you are menstruating, have high or low blood pressure, have a hernia or ulcer, have recently had abdominal illness or trauma, have glaucoma, suffer from heart disease, or are pregnant.

It's important to practice on an empty stomach, and ideally empty your bladder and bowels before starting. Learn each lock individually before trying to do them all the same time.

Throat Lock (Jalandhara Bandha)

The Throat Lock, or chin lock, restricts the upward flow of energy and usually also involves breath retention (holding your breath).

Sit in a meditative position. Your head, neck, and spine should be long and straight.

Take a deep breath in and at the same time elevate your sternum and rib cage slightly, bringing them closer to your chin.

Now, while holding your breath, lower your chin and jaw and place them onto your upper chest, right in the notch between your two collarbones. It will feel like you're trying to give yourself the appearance of a "double chin." If you can't touch your upper chest with your chin, you can place a rolled washcloth between your chin and chest.

Hold this position for a count of five, and then raise your head back to the starting position as you exhale.

Be careful that you don't tense your neck or tilt it to the side while performing the Throat Lock.

Root Lock (Mula Bandha)

The root of your body is your pelvic floor. This is a diamond-shaped area that contains your anus, genitals, and perineum (the ridged area between your anus and genitals). You achieve the Root Lock by pulling inward at the perineum. This probably sounds very vague, so let's go through it step-by-step.

Sit in a meditative position, with your spine long and straight, while gazing forward (you can also close your eyes if you wish).

Inhale and contract your entire pelvic floor by pulling it inward and upward. Exhale and slowly release the contraction. Repeat this a few times.

Now, practice these same contractions but reverse the breathing. So you'll contract on the exhalation and relax on the inhalation.

When you're comfortable with lifting your entire pelvic region upwards, you can focus on the specific area of your perineum.

You can isolate this area by using the same contraction you would if you were trying to hold in your urine. For women, it also helps to imagine that lifting sense you make when you're menstruating and want to stop leaking. This is how it feels to lock the mula bandha. If this doesn't work, you can also sit with your legs crossed and imagine you're levitating. That pulling upwards and contraction is your mula bandha activating.

Once you've found a way to isolate and contract your perineum, you can bring your breath into the practice.

Inhale and contract that area inward and upward. Exhale as you release.

Now, try to reverse your breathing again. Contract as you exhale and relax as you inhale.

Once you are able to manipulate the perineum and mula bandha with your breath, you will be able to train yourself to hold it for longer and longer periods of time. Try to eventually maintain the contraction as you continue to breathe for 10 breaths.

You'll also be naturally engaging mula bandha throughout your day without even realizing it. This happens when you climb stairs, ride a bike, or even while carrying your shopping bags. When you engage your Root Lock during your yoga practice (while doing certain poses), you'll allow your energy to flow up and not down. It leaves you with a "floaty" feeling. You'll have a sense of lightness and your body won't feel as heavy on the mat. Ideal poses to practice mula bandha are Tree Pose, Downward Facing Dog, and Bridge Pose.

Stomach Lock (Uddiyana Bandha)

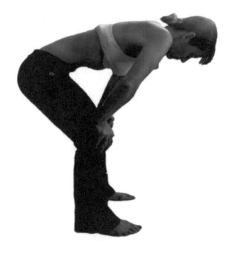

Uddiyana means to fly or rise up (Wortman, 2017). This is what you will be doing with your diaphragm. Essentially you will exhale and hold it there while pressing your abdominal wall inwards and drawing the contents upward. It produces a hollowing at the base of your rib cage and when you release this powerful contraction, your inhalation is automatically "sucked in." It's quite a remarkable feeling once you get it right, but it can be tricky in the beginning.

The easiest position to start with is to stand with your feet shoulder-width apart, bend your knees, and fold forward (keeping your back straight). Place your hands on your thighs. Keep your elbows straight and shift the weight of your upper body onto your arms.

Take a long, slow exhale and hold it there. For this lock, it helps to get as much air out as possible. Pretend you're blowing up a balloon as much as you can with one single breath.

Now, with a "false inhale"—the action of taking a breath without taking any air in—draw your abdomen in and up. You'll make an upward movement with your diaphragm and pull your organs up and towards your back. It helps to try to imagine pulling your waist in as much as you can to make it smaller and smaller.

To get the hang of the "false inhale" it helps to block your mouth and nose with your hands and breathe in. You should feel your chest lift. While holding the breath out, try harder to inhale while keeping your abdomen relaxed. This is important—you're not engaging your core or contracting your outer abdominal muscles. You're "sucking" your organs up.

When you get it right, your upper abdomen will form a deep hollow under your rib cage. That is uddiyana bandha. Hold it for a few seconds, then release your abdomen slowly.

Gently inhale, without gasping. You'll find that air is naturally sucked into your lungs again once you release the lock.

Breathe naturally and smoothly for a few moments and don't repeat more than twice.

The Stomach Lock moves energy upwards much more powerfully than mula bandha on its own. It massages the internal muscles in your lower back and is fantastic for digestive issues.

Combined Lock (Maha Bandha)

Once you have mastered each of the locks individually, you can try to combine them and do them all at the same time.

Stand with your feet about shoulder-width apart and your knees bent. Rest your hands on your thighs and keep your elbows straight.

Exhale slowly and hold your breath out.

Activate the Throat Lock and immediately contract your abdomen as you perform the Stomach Lock.

Once these are in place, activate the Root Lock.

Hold these locks together for three to five seconds.

Release them slowly and with control, in this specific order:

1. Release the contraction in your abdomen and let go of your Stomach Lock.

2. This release will weaken and release your Root Lock naturally.

3. Release the Throat Lock and breath in slowly. Make sure you've fully released your Root Lock.

4. Breathe naturally for a few moments and repeat only once or twice more.

If you feel pressure behind your eyes or in your temple area, or if your breathing is labored, then you have gone beyond your current capacity. You need to gradually work your way up to this advanced practice and only lengthen the time spent in this complete lock when your body allows you to do so comfortably.

Once you start practicing these three locks regularly, you'll start to notice subtle changes in your energy. This will be even more evident if you incorporate it into your yoga asana practice. Another more subtle way of harnessing energy is through mudras. We'll have a closer look at these hand seals in the next chapter.

Chapter 7:

Yoga In Your Hands

Mudra is a Sanskrit term that means seal or mark. Mudras are symbolic gestures you can perform with your hands and are often used during breathing exercises, meditation, and various yoga poses.

The theory behind mudras is that they guide the energy flow to specific parts of the brain, depending on the finger and hand placement, as well as their connection points.

The five universal elements are fire, air, water, earth, and ether. These are also present in each of our cells and every person has a unique combination of the elements. This is the foundation of *Ayurveda*, an ancient medicinal practice which has the goal of bringing a person to their unique balance of the elements.

When there is an imbalance of the elements, it can be experienced as disease in the body. Mudras are designed to recreate that equilibrium.

It is believed that each of the five fingers represents these elements. The thumb is fire and universal consciousness, the index finger is air and individual consciousness. The middle finger is akasha or connection, the ring finger is earth, and the pinky finger is water.

Different areas of the hands are connected with corresponding parts of the body and brain. When mudras are performed regularly, your brain makes connections and forms patterns. Eventually, unconscious reflexes take place in the brain as soon as your hands go into a specific shape. This, in turn, balances and redirects your body's internal energy and positively affects organs, muscles, tendons, and glands.

There are over 100 mudras used in yoga. We'll take a closer look at the most commonly used ones.

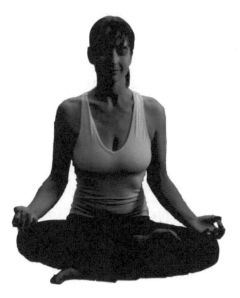

Mudra of Knowledge (Gyan Mudra)

This is one of the most well-known mudras and is often seen while in seated meditation or in Lotus Position. It's performed by touching the index finger against the thumb to form a closed circle, while keeping the other three fingers straight. It symbolizes the unity of fire and air, universal and individual consciousness.

The *gyan* mudra, also called the Chin Mudra or *jnana* mudra, is said to be connected to the root chakra and to reduce tension and depression. It is calming and spiritually awakening because it stimulates the air element. It is designed to increase concentration and creativity, as well as to sharpen the mind, minimizing stress and anger.

If you need to feel receptive and open, keep your palms facing upwards. If you need more grounding, rest your palms facing down on your legs.

Meditation Mudra (Dhyana Mudra)

You may recognize the *dhyana* mudra from an image of the Buddha, who was often pictured performing this mudra. It is meant to bring you into a deep sense of concentration and provides a feeling of inner peace.

It is done by simply sitting with your palms facing upward, right hand resting on top of the left. The right hand symbolizes enlightenment, and the left represents the world of illusion (also called *maya*).

Prayer Mudra (Anjali Mudra)

Anjali means "to offer" and is a gesture of openness and receptivity. This mudra is essentially your hands in Prayer Position at your sternum (commonly referred to as your "heart center"). It is often used at the beginning and end of practice, and during certain poses (such as Mountain Pose and Tree Pose).

Perhaps one of the most beautiful descriptions of the *anjali* mudra is by the yoga master, Krishnamacharya: "This gesture signifies the potential for an intention to progress to greatest spiritual awakening. When done properly the palms are not flat against each other; the knuckles at the base of the fingers are bent a little, creating space between the palms and fingers of the two hands resembling a flower yet to open, symbolizing the opening of our hearts" (*The Real Meaning of Anjali Mudra or "Prayer" Posture*, 2020).

Letting Go Mudra (Ksepana Mudra)

Ksepana mudra is a gesture that symbolizes letting go and pouring out. You use it when you feel like you need to release negative energy. It helps alleviate frustration and stress, and helps to re-establish positivity.

It can be practiced while seated or in poses that involve holding the arms above the head, such as in Warrior I.

You perform this mudra by interlacing your fingers and extending both your index fingers, and crossing your thumbs. This is the point where the negative energy can be focused out. Press your index fingers together and imagine bad thoughts leaving your body.

Lotus Mudra

The lotus mudra is connected to the heart and emotions and symbolizes purity and transformation. A lotus flower on the surface of a pond will open up its petals to the sun, while its roots remain firmly rooted in the muddy bottom. They grow from the murky depths and it symbolizes our ability to overcome obstacles and still remain soft and receptive. It's a beautiful image of light and beauty emerging from darkness.

To perform this mudra, start with your hands in Prayer at your heart center. Now, keeping the heels of your hands, thumbs, and pinky fingers touching, open up your remaining fingers to look like an open flower. Hold this mudra with your thumbs against your sternum.

Ganesh Mudra

Ganesh (also known as *Ganesha*) is a Hindu god with an elephant head on a man's body. This deity is considered the remover of all obstacles. The *ganesh* mudra can create feelings of warmth and safety, and is useful for easing symptoms of depression and feelings of heaviness. If you're struggling with a decision or feel blocked in some way, this is the perfect mudra to practice. The arms are positioned across the chest because often, the greatest obstacle we face is ourselves.

To perform this mudra, first bring the palms together in *anjali* mudra. Now, swivel your hands so that your fingertips point towards opposite elbows. The right palm will be facing your body and the left palm faces away. Once you have this right, slide your hands back until you're able to lock your fingers together and clasp your hands. Keep your hands at heart level.

It's quite a powerful mudra to use during breathing practices, such as the Breath of Fire (or Skull Shining Breath). If you're wondering what that is, read on. I'll be talking all about breathwork in the next chapter.

Chapter 8:

Breath Matters

You may remember the word Prana (life force) from an earlier chapter. We also spoke about the breath (*prana*) and how we can channel this energy in our bodies.

A new Sanskrit word I would like to introduce now is *yama*. This is translated as "control." When you combine the two words prana and yama you get *pranayama*, which is literally the act of controlling your breathing.

Pranayama channels energy through your body by using different breathing techniques. It is considered a physical and spiritual practice.

On a physical level, pranayama brings a larger supply of oxygen into the blood and oxygenates the entire body. Blood circulation improves and positively impacts the nerves, brain, spinal cord, and heart muscles.

A slow and steady breath reestablishes relaxed rhythms of the brain and heart rate. Conscious breathing also affects the expansion of your lungs and encourages the circulation of lymph and other fluids in your organs.

The rhythmic use of the diaphragm and abdominal muscles stimulates digestion and is a tremendous stress-reliever and improves concentration.

We'll now take a look at specific breathing techniques that you'll likely use in your yoga practice.

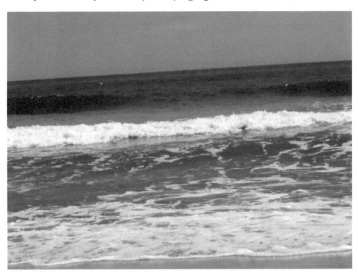

The Ocean Breath

The *ujjayi* breath, also known as the Ocean Breath, is a breathing technique often used during yoga classes. It helps to keep your breath smooth and rhythmic, and also allows you to keep your focus on your breathing in each pose. You'll find that by using this controlled breathing throughout your practice, you'll never be short of breath or find yourself holding your breath without realizing it. It keeps you constant, just like a metronome.

Ujjayi breathing is also called "victorious breathing" and sounds like wind through the trees or the gentle hum of the sea. It's regulated by breathing in and out through the nose with your lips sealed and activating the energy of the air in the back of your throat. It builds heat in your body and simultaneously relaxes and energizes your mind.

How to Perform the Ocean Breath

- Close your lips and breathe in and out through your nose.
- Your inhales will be slightly longer and deeper than usual and when you exhale, you'll contract the muscles in the back of your throat.
- If you're doing it correctly, the sound that is made in your throat (on the inhalation and exhalation) will sound like ocean waves or a gentle snore. The exhale will be a bit louder than the inhale.
- This breathing technique feels like a gentle stroke on the back of your throat.

To perfect the sound and sensation of the Ocean Breath, start by practicing it like this:

Open your mouth and pretend you're misting up a window. Now close your mouth and make the same sound as you breathe in and out.

You can also mimic the action of breathing in and out through a straw (with your lips open and around the "straw"). Now close your lips and breathe in the same way. Can you hear the ocean this time?

Once you've mastered the ocean breath you can start using it throughout your yoga practice, only returning to normal breathing when in Corpse Pose at the end.

Benefits of the Ocean Breath

This breathing technique balances the cardiovascular and respiratory systems and helps ease feelings of frustration. It calms your mind and body while building body heat and increasing the amount of oxygen in your blood.

Your energy flow will improve, helping regulate blood pressure and giving your yoga practice a distinct rhythm and sense of calm.

The ujjayi breath isn't just limited to the yoga studio, however. You can start regulating your breath this way when you feel stressed or agitated. It's particularly helpful for calming your nerves if you're feeling anxious.

Aerobic exercise such as running is more effective when you use the Ocean Breath to regulate the rhythm of your breath, helping you tire less easily.

The Square Breath

The Square Breath is incredible for anxiety, frustration, or when you're feeling overwhelmed. It calms you down and allows you to think more clearly. It also goes by its Sanskrit name, *Sama-Vritti Pranayama*.

While doing this breathing technique, you can use a soft and gentle Ocean Breath at the same time.

How to Perform the Square Breath

- Sit comfortably, with a straight spine, and bring awareness to your breath.
- Close your eyes.
- Inhale for a count of four, then hold your breath for a count of four.
- Exhale for a count of four, and hold your exhalation for another count of four.
- Repeat for as many times as you wish.

Bhramari Breath

Bhramari means "humming bee," and it refers to the sound you will make while performing this breathing technique.

How to Perform the Bhramari Breath

- Sit comfortably and close your eyes.
- Take a long, full exhale.
- You can engage Throat Lock (jalandara bhanda) if you wish.
- Inhale slowly and deeply through both nostrils.
- Exhale slowly and steadily until your lungs are completely empty while making a buzzing "mmmmmm" sound. Try and continue for 10 counts.
- Inhale again and return to normal breathing.

Variations

As you progress, you can make the sound louder and you can also do it through alternate nostrils.

You can include breath retentions after the inhalations or exhalations (or both).

Block your eyes and ears if you want a louder, more internal experience.

Benefits

Bhramari breathing is fantastic for improving focus, and the vibration is both stimulating and healing.

The vibration generated in the sinuses during exhalation produces nitric oxide. This promotes feelings of well-being and stimulates the parasympathetic nervous system. This helps you to relax and calms the body and mind.

The Bhramari Breath also stimulates the throat. This strengthens the voice and helps soothe a sore throat.

Avoid doing this one if you have an ear infection.

Alternate Nostril Breathing

This is a balancing breath and is believed to activate and balance the ida and pingala nadis. This balances the brain hemispheres and creates harmony in your thoughts. The breath is deep, but quiet.

Alternate nostril breathing brings equilibrium to the parasympathetic and sympathetic nervous systems. The nerves are calmed and the mind becomes lucid. It provides a great sense of peace, reduces stress, and improves sleep.

Alternate nostril breathing is known as *nadi shodona* in Sanskrit. Nadi, as we remember, means "energy channel" and *shodona* means "purifying."

How to Perform Alternate Nostril Breathing

- Sit comfortably with your spine straight and eyes closed.
- Place your fingertips on one side of your nose, and your thumb on the other side. They should be about halfway down your nose, just below the hard "notch."

- Keeping your nostrils open, just rest your fingers here with even pressure on both sides.
- Exhale the breath completely through both nostrils, then inhale through both nostrils.
- Block the right nostril and exhale slowly and completely out of the left.
- Empty your lungs completely.
- Inhale slowly and deeply through your left nostril, filling your lungs.
- Block your left nostril completely.
- Keeping the left nostril blocked, open the right one and exhale through it slowly and deeply.
- Empty your lungs completely.
- Inhale through the right nostril while keeping the left one blocked.
- Block your right nostril.
- Exhale through your left nostril completely.
- Repeat for a few rounds, ending by exhaling out of the left nostril.

Throughout alternate nostril breathing, it's important to make your exhalations and inhalations of equal duration.

Variations on Alternate Nostril Breathing

After you've mastered the standard method of performing alternate nostril breathing, you can start to retain the breath after inhalation by engaging Root Lock (mula bandha). Once you've managed to do this, you can practice retention of the breath after each exhalation and engaging Stomach Lock (uddiyana bandha).

The Cooling Breath

This breathing technique is also known as *sitali pranayama* in Sanskrit (*sital* means "cool"). It helps to cool down the body after a heated practice or a particularly hot day.

How to Perform the Cooling Breath

- Sit comfortably with a straight spine.
- Exhale your breath completely.
- Open your mouth and form an "o" shape with your lips.
- Curl the tongue up and protrude the curled up tongue through your lips.
- Inhale through your curled tongue and into the mouth while making a slurping sound to fill your lungs completely.
- If you can't curl your tongue (to make it look like a tube), you can purse your mouth with the tongue extended through the lips, and then draw the breath in as if you were drinking through a straw.
- Withdraw the tongue and close your mouth.
- Engage Throat Lock (jalandhara bandha) and exhale slowly through your nose.

- Repeat at least 10 times and finish the last breath by inhaling through your curled tongue and exhaling normally.

The Skull Shining Breath

This breathing technique is called *kapalabhati* in Sanskrit. *Kapala* means "skull" and *bhati* means "light." It is believed that the fluctuations in oxygen and energy levels in the mind during the Skull Shining Breath fills the mind with bright light and purifies the frontal lobe of the brain. It's also known as the "Breath of Fire."

During the Skull Shining Breath, your inhalation will be slow and passive, and your exhalations are vigorous and forced. After each exhalation there is also a split second of retention. The belly pumps back towards the spine on exhalation.

This breathing technique creates a core muscular contraction due to the diaphragm pumping up and down. It is an energizing breath that massages your organs and invigorates your liver, spleen, pancreas, and abdominal muscles. Naturally, this improves digestion. The Skull Shining Breath also stimulates cellular metabolism, strengthens your heart, and tones your organs.

The powerful exhales pump air out of the bottom of your lungs, forcing stale air out of your body, and this includes unwanted toxins. Your blood is purified and oxygen saturates your cells.

How to Perform the Skull Shining Breath

- Sit in a comfortable seat with your eyes closed.
- You can engage Throat Lock (jalandhara bandha) if you wish.
- Exhale completely.
- Inhale gently into your belly so that it expands slightly.
- Forcefully exhale, pumping the belly towards the back of your body.
- The inhale is slow and comes naturally due to the pressure difference created by the forceful exhalation.
- Continue to force the exhale (you're basically pumping the breath).
- Continue for 10 to 20 cycles.
- Finish with a long exhale.
- Repeat the whole exercise three times.

Variations on the Skull Shining Breath

You can practice the Skull Shining Breath while doing alternate nostril breathing.

This breathing technique must not be practiced if you're pregnant, or have any form of heart disease, high blood pressure, vertigo, epilepsy, history of stroke, panic disorder, hernia or gastric ulcers.

The Bellows Breath

The Bellows Breath is known as *bhastrika* (which literally means "bellows") in Sanskrit. It involves forceful breathing as if you were pumping the bellows of a blacksmith's fire. It's very similar to the Skull Shining Breath, but while that technique focuses on the exhalation, the Bellows Breath emphasizes both the inhalation and exhalation. They also differ in the length of the inhale. In the Skull Shining Breath, the exhale is longer, and the inhale is passive. Whereas in the Bellows Breath, both the inhalation and exhalation are the same length.

The Bellows Breath also goes by the nickname, "yogic coffee." It's stimulating and invigorating and provides a tremendous energy boost. It clears the mind, accelerates the metabolism, and improves digestion.

Some yoga texts state that this breathing technique cleanses the nadis and awakens Kundalini energy (Adele, 2019). It also helps to boost the immune system and can prevent colds by clearing nasal passages, sinuses, and lungs.

You may experience a sense of mild elation. Your heart rate will increase, and you'll feel your body warm up. This breath also helps relieve depression.

How to Perform the Bellows Breath

- Sit comfortably with a straight spine and with your shoulders relaxed.
- You can rest your hands on your belly.
- The first round begins on an inhale.
- Inhale and exhale rapidly through the nose. Your breaths need to be forceful. Use your diaphragm to pump your breath and feel your stomach move like a bellows beneath your hands.
- One inhale and exhales is one round of breath.
- Start by doing 10 rounds and see how you feel.
- After these 10 rounds, follow the last exhalation with a very deep inhalation. Hold this breath for as long as you can.
- Then slowly release the breath with a long, deep exhale.
- Breathe normally for a few minutes and then repeat the entire exercise three times.

Cautions With the Bellows Breath

As with the Skull Shining Breath, the Bellows Breath must be avoided if you are pregnant, or have any form of heart disease, high blood pressure, vertigo, epilepsy, history of stroke, panic disorder, hernia or gastric ulcers.

Because of the pumping action, you should never do this breathing technique on a full stomach—wait at least two hours after eating. It's also not recommended to perform this breath close to bedtime due to its energizing properties.

Incorporating Breath With Movement

In many types of yoga, such as Vinyasa, you will pair your breath with movement. Each pose will either be performed while inhaling or exhaling, and it can get confusing to know which happens when!

Once you are able to coordinate your breath with your movement, you will find that your practice flows and becomes meditative in nature.

Here are a few tips to make sure you're breathing correctly:

1. When you bend forward or fold over, exhale.

   As you breathe out, your lungs empty; this makes your torso more compact, deepening the fold.

2. When you open or expand the chest or raise your arms, inhale.

   Inhalations increase the space in your torso and fill you with air.

3. When doing a twist, exhale.

   You inhale as you prepare for the twist (such as lifting your arms), and then exhale as you twist around. You can imagine you're "squeezing air out" with the twist.

Remember that inhaling increases length and expands, while exhaling deepens folds and constricts the twist more.

If you do just one breath technique, connecting even basic inhales and exhales properly to flowing asana movements can be the most simple and powerful way to engage your breath in your yoga practice.

In an upcoming chapter, we'll put this all together with guided sequences. I'll guide you through the poses, and include cues on when to inhale and when to exhale. Eventually, it will come naturally!

Chapter 9:

Find Your Focus

The beautiful, inspiring, healing practice of Eye Gazes (Drishti) involves looking toward a particular body part or outward direction for the duration of a pose or breathing practice. Drishti means focus, gaze or vision. Drishti to some degree relates to all eight limbs of yoga, mentioned earlier in this book, but most directly relates to the practice of pratyahara (sensory withdrawal), and dharana (concentration). If feeling restless or distracted is a challenge for you when practicing yoga, incorporating Drishti may be a curative next step.

Drishti (Eye Gaze) practice creates a one-pointed focus that can help to still and calm the mind during asana practice (poses) or during pranayama (breathwork). Drishti, through a single physical focus, can create a unified mental focus. Drishti is particularly helpful for balance poses.

Practicing Eye Gazes can turn your yoga practice into a moving meditation. You can also think of it as focus training. The inwardness, stillness and steady focus offered by Drishti practice can dramatically increase the mental benefits of your yoga practice.

Incorporating Eye Gazes can enable you to focus less on random thoughts and more on your inner body experiences during your yoga practice. Drishti practice is a way to think more clearly, have more discipline in your focus and thoughts, and have less mental fatigue. Drishti also has more esoteric functions that we will touch on later in this chapter.

To practice Drishti, choose a single focal point for each pose or breathing exercise. Look in one direction with your eyes, and endeavor to keep your gaze fixed until you shift out of that pose or breathing practice.

Use a soft gaze, perhaps with your eyes half closed, making sure never to strain your eyes. Keep the muscles of your forehead and around your eyes relaxed. If you find you have moved your gaze while still in a pose, or find your eyes wandering, simply notice this, and return to the Eye Gaze.

Stick with one Eye Gaze for the duration of one pose. When you change poses, switch to the appropriate Drishti for the following pose by shifting where you look as you move from one pose to the next.

Some of the most commonly used Eye Gazes (Drishti), along with applicable poses and breathing practices are listed below. Some poses harmonize with more than one

Drishti, although it is best to stick with one for the duration of a practice.

1. **Toes Gaze (Padayoragrai Drishti)** Look toward the toes. This helps to lengthen the spine and extend the energy deeper into the pose: Seated Forward Fold, Standing Forward Fold, most forward folds.

2. **Thumbs Gaze (Angusthamadhye Drishti)** Gaze to the thumbs between the middle joint and the thumbnail: Upward Salute Pose, Chair Pose.

3. **Hand Gaze (Hastagrai Drishti)** Gaze to the hand or hands: Triangle Pose, Extended Side Angle Pose, Warrior One Pose, Reverse Warrior (gaze toward the upward hand).

4. **Navel Gaze (Nabi Chakra Drishti)** Gaze to the navel. This Drishti is sometimes called the magic circle: Downward Facing Dog Pose, Bridge Pose, Shoulder Stand.

5. **Backward Gaze (Parsva Drishti)** Gaze as far back as you can behind you to the right or left side, sometimes referred to as two separate Drishti based on whether facing left or right: twist poses.

6. **Upward Gaze (Urdhva Drishti)** Sometimes called Outward Gaze or Skyward Gaze. Look up as if into infinity: Warrior One Pose, Warrior Two Pose, Half Moon Pose.

7. **Tip of the Nose Gaze (Nasagrai Drishti)** Gaze down toward the tip of your nose: Plank Pose, Upward Facing Dog, Standing Forward Fold, Easy Pose, Lotus Pose, Cat/Cow Pose, Tree Pose (You can also look to a steady spot nearby.), Cobra Pose, Dancer's Pose, any sort of back bend. Tip of the Nose Gaze is also another option for forward folds.

8. **Third Eye Gaze (Bhrumadhye Drishti)** Gaze between and above the eyebrows. Eyes can be half open or closed: Pose of a Child, Easy Pose, Corpse Pose, and during many breathing practices (pranayama.)

Pay attention to the alignment of your spine and neck as you gaze. Do not reach excessively with your neck and head toward the focal point. Remember, as always, to breathe.

You may notice that one of these Eye Gazes is not a commonly understood body part or direction, and is instead someplace you cannot actually see through your visual gaze. This Eye Gaze (Drishti) is the Third Eye Gaze (Bhrumadhye Drishti). Have you seen pictures of Indian people with a dot of color or a shiny stuck-on bead between their eyebrows? This is not simply a fashion statement; this is also a way of honoring the Third Eye.

To apply this Drishti, imagine that instead of looking out through your eyes, you are lifting up from your eyeballs to inside your head, as if you are looking out from between and slightly above your eyebrows. Rather than an actual gaze, the Third Eye Gaze creates a sense of gazing from this spiritually and hormonally potent location above and between the eyes.

Sitting essentially at the center of the brain, the Third Eye is also the location of the pineal gland. The pineal gland directs your sleep and wakefulness cycles by regulating melatonin production. It also influences sexual development, healthy menstruation, antioxidant usage, production of healthy cells (think anti-cancer), heart health, blood pressure, mood regulation, and the immune system (Healthline 2017, Michael 2019). In some animals, the fascinating pineal gland also plays a role in hibernation and migration.

There are some who say the Third Eye is the true place where your left eye vision and right eye vision unite. This point is sometimes called the eye of the mind or the connection point with a higher power. However you choose to think of the Third Eye, using this Eye Gaze can have a powerful impact.

If you dislike working with the Third Eye Gaze, or it just feels like too much, look instead straight ahead at a fixed point in the space where you are practicing. You can also look to the tip of your nose. Later, when you have practiced yoga using less intense drishtis for a while, perhaps when you feel that your monkey mind is quiet more often as you practice, then you can revisit the Third Eye Gaze practice.

Once you are familiar with the basic patterns of Eye Gazes, it becomes fairly intuitive to know where it is best to look while practicing most poses. As a rule of thumb, choose a Drishti in each pose that focuses in the direction of the stretch.

A supported way to start practicing Drishti is to sit in Easy Pose, light a candle at about eye level in front of you, and stare at the flame while you breathe.

Drishti should be calming and focusing, not causing strain and struggle. If you cannot gaze all the way up to your hands or all the way down to your toes, gaze part way up or down. If you cannot gaze without eye strain all the way to the back of the room as you twist, gaze wherever you can with gentle effort. If gazing at the tip of the nose feels too challenging, gaze instead straight in front of you or down to the front edge of your mat. If gazing at your uplifted hands is too much, gaze at some fixed point in space slightly upward. You can also blink several times or briefly rest your eyes closed.

If you become dizzy at any point, drop into Pose of a Child with eyes closed until the dizziness subsides.

If you find Eye Gazes challenging to the point that your practice feels stressful, postponing Drishti practice may be the best choice for you.

It is okay to choose whatever Eye Gaze supports you to feel relaxed, aligned, and invigorated in the pose. It is more important that you pick a single point of focus than it is that you practice the Drishti in its full, traditional expression. As long as you are holding a fixed, relaxed, alignment-supportive gaze in each pose, you are doing it right.

I encourage you, as you embark on this impactful yoga habit, to honor that for some, Drishti practice brings esoteric benefits, such as getting in touch with your own soul or with higher levels of consciousness. If this sounds far-fetched to you, focus more on Drishti's straightforward benefits, such as more organized thinking and better concentration.

Have you ever noticed that babies are great at staring, at their own toes or at some random spot in the room? Eye Gazes, like many yogic habits, support you to reconnect with the simple, quiet presence from within.

Eye Gaze practice can free you from some of your emotional armor and prejudices from past experience, and can help you to release reactiveness that sometimes can overtake more thoughtful responses to life's challenges. Through the singular focus of Drishti practice, you can learn to prioritize your attention on and off the mat.

Drishti practice can offer a path to the core of who you are inside. Through the focused limits of Drishti, you may find a sense of connecting with your intrinsic, innocent witness to life, or perhaps the wise, unlimited old soul within. This can make an enormous difference in how you feel, how you practice yoga, and how you respond to the outward conditions of your life.

Chapter 10:

Putting It Into Practice

Now that you have learned some key poses and other vital yoga habits, you may be wondering how to put it all together. Transitions between postures are just as important as the poses themselves, and the flow needs to be graceful, intelligent, and aligned.

The most important things to remember, if you're ever setting up your own sequences, is the following:

- Everything you do on one side needs to be duplicated on the other side (this ensures balance and alignment).
- If you do a backbend, you should counteract it with some form of forward fold.
- Start with simple, warm-up poses, then work your way up to a strong flow.
- Finish with some kind of rest pose.

I've included three full sequences for you to start off with. Each one has a strong intention, an intelligent and natural flow, and includes poses that we've covered in this book.

Once you are comfortable with these sequences, you can start adding extra asanas into the flow to make them longer. Gradually, you can work your way up to designing your own sequences completely.

"I am Strong" Sequence

This is a sequence designed to make you feel focused, strong, and self-aware. You can set your intention or mantra before you start. Remember your chosen phrase throughout your practice. Here are a few suggestions:

- I am strong.
- I am powerful.
- I can do anything I set my mind to.
- I am capable.
- I am fierce.

Your Strong Flow

1. Start in Plank Pose. Try to hold it for at least five breaths.

2. On an exhale, move into Downward Facing Dog. Once again, hold this pose for five breaths.

3. Inhale and raise your right leg to the sky (Three-Legged Dog), then exhale as you step your right foot between your hands.

4. Inhale and stand up into high lunge (this is the same as Warrior I but with your hands at heart center not above your head). Stay here for five breaths.

5. Exhale and enter Warrior II pose. Gaze over your front fingers and remember your mantra. Hold for five breaths.

6. Shift into Reverse Warrior and hold for a count of two.

7. Swivel your torso as you lift your left leg, transitioning into Warrior III. See if you can hold this for three to five breaths.

8. Bring your left foot forward and seat yourself into Chair Pose. Hold for five breaths. If you prefer to not have your hands raised above your head, you may choose to hold them in a mudra instead. Good examples include holding your hands in lotus mudra or anjali mudra as you hold strong in Chair Pose.

9. Straighten your legs and bend over into Standing Forward Fold. Let it all go, remember your intention, and stay here for a count of five breaths.

10. Step back into Plank Pose and hold again for five breaths.

11. Exhale and lower down to Low Plank (Chaturanga), and on your next inhale, move to Upward Facing Dog.

12. Exhale to Downward Facing Dog and hold for five breaths. Now you'll repeat this on the other side.

13. Inhale and raise your left leg to the sky (Three-Legged Dog), then exhale as you step your left foot between your hands.

14. Inhale and stand up into High Lunge and stay here for five breaths.

15. Exhale and enter Warrior II pose. Gaze over your front fingers and remember your mantra. Hold for five breaths.

16. Shift into Reverse Warrior and hold for a count of two.

17. Swivel your torso as you lift your right leg, transitioning into Warrior III. Hold for the same number of breaths you did on the other side.

18. Bring your right foot forward and seat yourself into Chair Pose (with or without your chosen mudra). Hold for five breaths.

19. Straighten your legs and bend over into Standing Forward Fold. Let it all go, remember your

intention, and stay here for a count of five breaths.

20. Step back into Plank Pose and hold again for five breaths.

21. Exhale and lower down to chaturanga (Low Plank), and on your next inhale, move to Upward Facing Dog.

22. Exhale to Downward Facing Dog.

23. Bring your knees to the floor and rest in Child's Pose.

"Time to Invigorate" Sequence

This sequence is designed to energize your mind and body, and is ideal to do in the mornings upon waking. Once again, consider setting an intention before you start. Here are some ideas:

- I feel alive.
- I am full of energy.
- I feel invigorated.
- I am ready for whatever comes my way.

Your Invigorating Sequence

1. Start in Tabletop Position and then do three rounds of cat/cow pose.

2. On an exhalation, move into Downward Facing Dog. Stay here for five breaths.

3. Step your feet between your hands and exhale as you fold forward. Once again, let it all go as you stay here for five breaths. Just breathe and release.

4. Inhale and raise your arms up to mountain pose. Gaze up at your hands and then on an exhale bring your hands down to the heart center (you can choose to place your palms together in anjali mudra if you so desire).

5. Proceed to Tree Pose, remembering to repeat the action on both left and right sides. Hold the pose for at least five breaths on each side.

6. Return to Mountain Pose with arms at your heart center in Prayer, close your eyes and recenter. Take your time here.

7. On an exhale fold forward, and then step your left foot back, and come up to Warrior II. Hold it steady for a count of five breaths.

8. Move into reverse warrior, and then flow into Extended Side Angle.

9. Place your hands on the mat on either side of your right foot. Step back into Downward Facing Dog. Stay here for five breaths.

10. Step your left foot forward and rise up to Warrior II. Hold it here for five breaths. Remember to repeat your intention or mantra.

11. Move into reverse warrior, and move into Extended Side Angle.

12. Place your hands on the mat on either side of your left foot. Step back into Downward Facing Dog. Hold for five breaths.

13. Step your feet between your hands and exhale as you move into Standing Forward Fold. Sigh out a long exhale and give yourself some time here.

14. Raise your hands as you inhale and transition to Chair Pose. Hold for a count of five breaths.

15. Exhale as you fold forward.

16. Step back into plank, hold for a count of three, and then exhale to Low Plank (Chaturanga).

17. Allow your belly to sink all the way to the ground and inhale for Cobra Pose. Hold Cobra for five breaths.

18. Place your hands beneath your shoulders and come to Tabletop Position, then raise your hips to the sky and shift into Downward Facing Dog. Hold once again for five breaths.

19. Bring your knees to the floor again and transition into Child's Pose. Allow yourself to rest here for five breaths.

20. Roll onto your back and proceed to do Bridge Pose. If you're feeling comfortable and strong enough, you can do Shoulder Stand here instead. Hold for 10 breaths.

21. Lower back down to your mat and bring your knees to your chest as a recovery pose. Give yourself a nice, long hug.

22. Come to a seated position and extend your legs straight out in front of you, moving into a Seated Forward Fold. Bend your legs generously if you need. Stay here for a count of five breaths.

23. Finally, lie down in Corpse Pose and linger here for as long as you need.

"Come Into Alignment" Sequence

This sequence is created to bring your body into alignment and to stretch sore muscles. It builds strength, stability, and stamina. It's a fantastic stress-reliever and restores confidence.

Here are some affirmations to use throughout the flow:

- I feel balanced.
- I am secure.
- I feel aligned and connected.
- I am a conqueror.

Your Aligned Sequence

1. Start in Mountain Pose with your eyes closed. Set your intention and repeat your chosen affirmation. Stay here for at least five breaths.

2. Inhale and raise your hands to upward salute (this is also known as High Mountain).

3. Step your left foot back into Warrior I (your right leg will be bent in front) and hold for a count of five breaths.

4. Swivel on your hips as you shift into Warrior II, once again holding for five counts.

5. Straighten your front leg and move into triangle pose and hold for three to five breaths.

6. Bend your right leg and transition to Extended Side Angle.

7. Windmill your hands down to the mat on either side of your right foot. Step your right foot back to Downward Facing Dog. Hold this for at least five breaths.

8. Step your left foot forward and rise into Warrior I on the left side. Hold for a count of five breaths.

9. Swivel on your hips as you shift into Warrior II, once again holding for five counts.

10. Straighten your front leg and move into Triangle Pose and hold for three to five breaths.

11. Bend your left leg and transition to Extended Side Angle.

12. Windmill your hands down to the mat on either side of your left foot. Step your left foot back to Downward Facing Dog. Hold this for at least five breaths. ·

13. Walk your hands forward and lower yourself into Plank. Hold for five breaths.

14. Lower your belly to the mat and proceed to Cobra Pose.

15. Finally, push back into Child's Pose and stay here for as long as you need.

When you've reached your resting poses at the end of your sequences, which are usually Corpse Pose or Child's Pose, you may wish to do a guided meditation or visualization. This helps to integrate your practice and is a beautiful way to reward yourself for all your hard work. In the next chapter, I'll guide you through such a meditation.

Yoga Made Simple

If you are not feeling ready for the complexity of all that yoga has to offer, for lifestyle reasons, medical reasons, due to overwhelm, or any other reason that makes figuring out how to navigate even a beginner's version of a fuller yoga practice feel like too much, you can simply do the following:

1. Learn and regularly practice Sun Salutation A. Repeat the Sun Salutation A short series of linked poses a minimum of 3 times during each practice.

2. Learn Ocean Breath while just sitting and breathing.

3. Practice doing Ocean Breath as you move through your sun salutations. Remember the rule of thumb that you inhale as you expand or raise up and exhale as you fold or contract. Move through the poses at the pace of your own Ocean Breath.

4. Try to do Root Lock (Mula Bandha), especially during downward dog. You may not feel it working, but don't be discouraged! It takes time.

   Try every day to pull your belly button back towards your spine and up towards your head with each inhale during down dog. Picture a hammock or satchel containing your whole lower belly cavity, pulled together back and up your spine, lifting ever so slightly. Then, strive to hold that lock during exhalation.

   If doing this is causing you to chest breathe, then try instead to pull your belly in and back slowly on exhales. Reread the Root Lock (Mula Bandha) section of this book a few times as you try to grasp the process.

5. Do Corpse Pose (Savasana) or Pose of a Child (Balasana) for at least one minute after you complete your Sun Salutations for the day.

That is it!

When you are ready to advance, add in three or more daily rounds of Sun Salutation B. Chair pose is also a great time to work on Root Lock.

If Root Lock or even Ocean Breath are overwhelming you, skip them at first. Do return to them when you can. For now, just think of using your core strength and breathing deeply instead.

This may not seem like much of a practice, but you will be amazed by how transformative this tiny bit of yoga can be if practiced regularly. Later, if you advance your practice, you can always return to this ultra-simple yoga habit on days when it is all you have time for, or otherwise seems best for you.

Chapter 11:

Bonus Guided Visualization

This chapter includes a 10-minute-long meditation and visualization that can be used while in Rest Pose at the end of your yoga practice, whenever you need to calm your anxiety, or perhaps just to start your day.

Meditation is not trying to stop our thoughts, but rather observing them. You simply watch them come and go. This guided meditation will help you do that.

If you do not have the audiobook version of this book, I suggest you record yourself reading this meditation out loud. I'll mention where you need to be silent for a set period of time. Then, once you have it recorded, you can simply play it back to yourself whenever you need the guidance. Read slowly and clearly, with a soft voice.

Guided Meditation

Lie down or find a comfortable seat. Make sure you're warm enough and do all the movements you need to before settling in.

Close your eyes and take three deep breaths in through the nose and out through the mouth.

Inhale. Breathe into your chest and belly, your ribs, and your back. Feel the cool air against your nostrils.

Exhale. Let it all go with an audible sigh.

Inhale. Fill your lungs and feel the air expand throughout your body.

Exhale. Release.

Inhale deeply through your nose.

And exhale, sigh it all out.

Now return to your regular breath in and out through the nose.

Check in with your environment. Notice any sounds around you. It could be noises in the street, or a bird outside your window. You may simply hear the sound of your own breath. Take in all the sounds. Become aware of each one.

If any thoughts enter your mind, allow them to be there. Observe them. Then watch them leave again. Don't pay any attention to the details of the thought, just watch it move through your mind.

Return to the sounds. Focus on everything you can hear.

Now 30 seconds of silence.

Now start to notice the sensations on your skin. Feel your body against your mat or the chair. Feel the weight of your organs and even down to the subtleties such as your heart beating, and your blood flowing through your veins. Can you feel the air against your skin? Come back to your breath and feel the cool air enter your nose when you inhale, and the warm air as you exhale.

Once again, if thoughts come and go, let them be. Just keep returning to the sensations in your body, and the feeling of your chest rising and falling as you breathe.

Now 30 seconds of silence.

Now scan your body and feel each body part as you go. We'll start with the soles of your feet. Concentrate on the sole of your left foot. Now turn your attention to your right sole.

Your left big toe, second toe, third toe, fourth toe, baby toe.

Your right big toe, second toe, third toe, fourth toe, baby toe.

The top of your left foot, your left ankle, your left calf.

The top of your right foot, your right ankle, your right calf.

Your left knee.

Remember to breathe. Inhale. Exhale.

Allow thoughts to come and go.

Your right knee.

The front of your left thigh, the back of your left thigh.

The front of your right thigh, the back of your right thigh.

Your hips. Swirl your attention around your pelvis and your hip bones.

Feel your glutes against your mat or the chair.

Settle into your abdomen and feel your organs. Notice as your stomach rises and falls with your breath.

Don't just think about your body, really feel it. Tune into the sensations.

Now move your attention to your rib cage. Your chest. Your diaphragm moving up and down.

Now to the back of your chest, your shoulder blades against the mat.

Feel your breath fill your lungs as you inhale, and feel them contract as you exhale.

Now move your attention down your left upper arm, your elbow, your forearm.

Feel it settle in your left wrist and move down your fingers. Your left thumb, forefinger, middle finger, ring finger, pinky finger.

Now move down your right arm, right elbow, and forearm. Feel your attention hover and settle around your wrist and then move towards your fingers. Your right thumb, forefinger, middle finger, ring finger, pinky finger.

Shift your attention to your neck and notice if you're holding any tension there. Let it go with your breath. Move up the back of your head and feel your skull, the hair on your head.

Your left ear, right ear.

Your jaw, lips, tongue, teeth.

Your nose. Your left cheek, right cheek.

Your left eye. Your right eye.

Your forehead.

Can you sense your third eye, that point between your eyebrows?

Focus on the top of your head and take a long, slow exhale.

Now 30 seconds of silence.

Focus on your breath now.

Breathe in for a count of four.

One, two, three, four.

Hold the air in your lungs for a count of four.

One, two, three, four.

Exhale. One, two, three, four.

Hold. One, two, three, four.

Let's do that a few more times.

Inhale. One, two, three, four.

Hold. One, two, three, four.

Exhale. One, two, three, four.

Hold. One, two, three, four.

Inhale. One, two, three, four.

Hold. One, two, three, four.

Exhale. One, two, three, four.

Hold. One, two, three, four.

Inhale. One, two, three, four.

Hold. One, two, three, four.

Exhale. One, two, three, four.

Hold. One, two, three, four.

Inhale. One, two, three, four.

Hold. One, two, three, four.

Exhale. One, two, three, four.

Hold. One, two, three, four.

Inhale. One, two, three, four.

Hold. One, two, three, four.

Exhale. One, two, three, four.

Hold. One, two, three, four.

Last round.

Inhale. One, two, three, four.

Hold. One, two, three, four.

Exhale. One, two, three, four.

Hold. One, two, three, four.

Return to your normal breathing and bring your awareness to your thoughts. Look at your thoughts as if you were an outside observer or witness. Watch yourself thinking the thoughts. You are not your thoughts or your emotions. You simply are. You're an observer.

Watch them come and watch them go.

Remember to breathe.

Simply be aware of what is happening inside, with no judgment, and no interference. Just see.

Now 30 seconds of silence.

Now, bring your awareness back to the present moment, still with your eyes closed. Imagine the room around you. Feel the sensations in your body, maybe rub your fingers together and wiggle your toes.

Feel the weight of your body on your mat and the temperature of the air on your skin.

Take in all the sounds around you and take a deep breath in, and a deep breath out.

When you're ready, you can slowly open your eyes.

Chapter 12:

Your Personal Best

The Best Yogis

Who are the best yogis? There are certainly renowned yogis and yoginis. There may also be that person with the most amazing-looking practice that you see on a nearby mat when you are in yoga class, or in an online video. Certainly, their powerful asana practice can be linked to embodying what yoga is, at a high level. Maybe they even showcase deep awareness and capacity for all eight limbs. Yet it is important to keep in mind that measuring success in yoga is not the same as measuring success in, say, tennis, or even Pilates.

Yoga is integrally designed to meet you where you are today, in this moment. Yoga practice is a combination of guiding your body into progressing in the poses, while also trying to hear what you and your body need. Some days your best practice might be to do fewer poses, or to modify them. When you do this, you are doing the best yoga. If your yoga practice is good for you, brings you benefits, and is not adding to your hurts, then *you* are the best yogi. The spirit of yoga is not to look the best or even meet a particular goal, but instead to have the practice support the care of you and your self-development.

The Best Yoga Teachers

Who are the best yoga teachers? You have already figured out from the last section that this is sort of a trick question, right?

The best yoga teacher is different for each person and can even change at different phases of your yoga journey. To dictate what is best in general in a yoga teacher is tricky. This may have been somewhat easier to define in the local Indian culture of yoga's birth and early development. Although, even there, many schools of thought existed. With yoga's current global reach and the variety of physical, emotional, cultural, social, and spiritual needs of yoga practitioners, any hard and fast definition would surely fall short.

Yoga, by its essence, is designed to meet the student where they need to be met. This is why all the variations in how people practice and teach are difficult to judge from an outside standard. A great yoga teacher might only be right for a few people. This does not diminish the greatness of what they offer to their students. So, ask not, "who are the best yoga teachers?" Ask instead, "who is the right yoga teacher for me at this time?" Be open to finding one lifelong teacher or many.

Having said that, some qualities to look for in a good teacher could include awareness of alignment, inclusion of breathing techniques, and kindness. If you are doing yoga prior to planning to get pregnant, make sure you are studying the bandhas, especially mula bandha.

I personally have had one teacher who has always felt like my most important teacher. Yet I have also learned invaluable lessons and experienced profound growth from contact with other teachers.

Your path in this regard is unique to you. I encourage you to listen deep within as you ponder these choices regarding your yoga habit.

Even the best teachers and most truly advanced yoga practitioners may, like all of us, have things to learn. Never forget that teachers frequently also learn from their students.

While I am here with you in a sense, as you read this book, and certainly do have your best interest in mind, working with this book does not constitute having a yoga teacher. This book will help you, I hope, to get started with yoga, and embrace a self-practice. Yet it is valuable, if you continue with your yoga habit, that you get feedback from a teacher who sometimes actually *sees* your practice (even if only on zoom.)

"When the student is ready, the teacher appears... When truly ready, the student becomes the teacher." – may be attributed to Buddha.

Conclusion

My wish and prayer is that your yoga journey is beautiful and ever-evolving. It's been an absolute privilege to share this time with you.

I would like to end with this blessing by Mike Heron (Thomsen, n.d.):

"May the long-time sun shine upon you

All love surround you

May the pure light within you

Guide Your Way On."

The light within me honors the light within you.

Appendix:

An A to Z of Yoga Poses

It would be impossible to cover all the yoga poses in one book, and although there are hundreds of asanas and variations, I have included a list of ones you are likely to come across during a class.

I provide the English and Sanskrit names, as well as the pose type. When you are setting up your own sequences and need a chest opener, for instance, you can run your finger down this list and find one that fits that description.

English	Sanskrit	Type of Pose
Seated or Low on the Mat		
Bharadvaja's Twist	Bharadvajasana I	Hip-Opening Seated Twist
Boat Pose	Paripurna Navasana	Core Seated Strengthening
Bound Angle	Baddha Konasana	Forward bend

Pose		Hip-Opening Seated
Cat Pose	Marjaryasana	Core
Child's Pose	Balasana	Forward Bend Hip-Opening Restorative
Corpse Pose	Savasana	Restorative
Cow Face Pose	Gomukhasana	Hip-Opening Seated
Easy Pose	Sukhasana	Hip-Opening Seated
Puppy Pose	Uttana Shishosana	Forward bend
Half Lord of the Fishes Pose	Ardha Matsyendrasana	Hip-Opening Seated Twist
Happy Baby Pose	Ananda Balasana	Core
Head-to-Knee Forward Bend	Janu Sirsasana	Forward bend Seated
Hero Pose	Virasana	Seated
Lotus Pose	Padmasana	Seated
Monkey Pose	Hanumanasana	Seated
Legs-Up-the-Wall Pose	Viparita Karani	Restorative
Plow Pose	Halasana	Inversion
Reclining Bound Angle Pose	Supta Baddha Konasana	Hip-Opening Restorative
Reclining Hand-to-Big-Toe Pose	Supta Padangusthasana	Restorative
Reclining Hero Pose	Supta Virasana	Restorative

Revolved Head-to-Knee Pose	Parivrtta Janu Sirsasana	Seated Twist
Seated Forward Bend	Paschimottanasana	Forward bend Seated
Staff Pose	Dandasana	Seated
Wide-Angle Seated Forward Bend	Upavistha Konasana	Forward Bend Hip-Opening Seated
Standing		
Big Toe Pose	Padangusthasana	Forward bend Standing Balance
Chair Pose	Utkatasana	Core Standing Strengthening
Dolphin Pose	Makarasana	Core Standing Strengthening
Downward-Facing Dog	Adho Mukha Svanasana	Forward bend Standing Strengthening
Hand-To-Big-Toe Pose	Utthita Hasta Padangustasana	Balancing Hip-Opening Standing
Extended Side Angle Pose	Utthita Parsvakonasana	Standing Strengthening
Triangle Pose	Utthita Trikonasana	Standing Strengthening
Garland Pose	Malasana	Standing
Gate Pose	Parighasana	Standing
High Lunge	Ashta Chandrasana	Standing

High Crescent Lunge	Anjaneyasana	Standing
Intense Side Stretch Pose	Parsvottanasana	Forward bend Standing
Low Lunge	Anjaneyasana	Standing
Mountain Pose	Tadasana	Standing
Revolved Side Angle Pose	Parivrtta Parsvakonasana	Standing Strengthening Twist
Revolved Triangle Pose	Parivrtta Trikonasana	Standing Strengthening Twist
Forward Fold	Uttanasana	Forward bend Standing
Standing Splits	Urdhva Prasarita Eka Padasana	Forward bend Standing
Upward Salute	Urdhva Hastasana	Standing
Warrior I Pose	Virabhadrasana I	Standing Strengthening
Warrior II Pose	Virabhadrasana II	Standing Strengthening
Warrior III Pose	Virabhadrasana III	Balancing Standing Strengthening
Wide-Legged Forward Bend	Prasarita Padottanasana	Forward bend Hip-Opening Standing Strengthening
Backbend		
Bow Pose	Dhanurasana	Chest-Opening Backbend

Bridge Pose	Setu Bandha Sarvangasana	Backbend
Camel Pose	Ustrasana	Chest-Opening Backbend
Cobra Pose	Bhujangasana	Chest-Opening Backbend
Cow Pose	Bitilasana	Chest-Opening Backbend
Fish Pose	Matsyasana	Chest-Opening Backbend
Half Frog Pose	Ardha Bhekasana	Chest-Opening Backbend
Locust Pose	Salabhasana	Chest-Opening Strengthening Backbend
One-Legged King Pigeon Pose	Eka Pada Rajakapotasana	Hip-Opening Backbend
Pigeon Pose	Kapotasana	Backbend
Sphinx Pose	Salamba Bhujangasana	Chest-Opening Backbend
Wheel Pose	Urdhva Dhanurasana	Chest-Opening Strengthening Backbend
Upward-Facing Dog Pose	Urdhva Mukha Svanasana	Chest-Opening Backbend
Balances		
Crane (Crow) Pose	Bakasana	Arm Balance Core
Dancer's Pose	Natarajasana	Balancing Chest-Opening Standing

		Backbend
Eagle Pose	Garudasana	Balancing Hip-Opening Standing
Eight-Angle Pose	Astavakrasana	Arm Balance
Firefly Pose	Tittibhasana	Arm Balance
Low Plank	Chaturanga Dandasana	Arm Balance Core Strengthening
Half Moon Pose	Ardha Chandrasana	Balancing Standing
Handstand	Adho Mukha Vrksasana	Balancing Inversion Strengthening
Peacock Pose	Mayurasana	Arm Balance
Plank Pose	Kumbhakasana	Arm Balance Core Strengthening
Side Crow Pose	Parsva Bakasana	Arm Balance
Side Plank Pose	Vasisthasana	Arm Balance Balancing Core
Headstand	Sirsasana	Balancing Inversion
Shoulderstand	Sarvangasana	Balancing Inversion
Tree Pose	Vrksasana	Balancing Standing
Wild Thing	Camatkarasana	Arm Balance Chest-Opening

References

A Brief History of Yoga. (2020, August 6). Art of Living (United States). https://www.artofliving.org/us-en/yoga/yoga-for-beginners/brief-history-yoga

Adele, T. (2019, August 30). *Need a Quick Energy Boost? Try This Energizing Breathing Technique (AKA Bellows Breath).* YogiApproved™. https://www.yogiapproved.com/yoga/bellows-breath-bhastrika/#:~:text=Bhastrika%20(Bellows%20Breath)%20is%20very

Eisler, M. (2016, January 29). *Learn the Ujjayi Breath, an Ancient Yogic Breathing Technique.* Chopra. https://chopra.com/articles/learn-the-ujjayi-breath-an-ancient-yogic-breathing-technique

Gendry, S. (2012, December 19). *Every Little Cell In My Body Is Happy.* American School of Laughter Yoga. https://www.laughteryogaamerica.com/sing/cell-body-happy-2-2944.php

Griffin, K. (2013, July 31). *21 Health Benefits of Yoga | How Yoga Improves Health and Wellness.* Yoga Journal. https://www.yogajournal.com/lifestyle/health/womens-health/good/

Healthline, (2017, April 7). *Five Functions of the Pineal Gland. https://www.healthline.com/health/pineal-gland-function*

Helfer, F. (2019, August 19). *How to Use a Yoga Strap: 18 Yoga Strap Stretches for Beginners*. Yoga Rove. https://yogarove.com/yoga-strap-stretches-beginners/

Instagram, A., & Twitter, A. (2021, April 22). *Sun Salutations Explained—and Why You Should Master Them*. Byrdie. https://www.byrdie.com/sun-salutation

Living, R. (2018, July 12). *A Short History of Yoga in India*. Replenish Yoga & Wellness | International Falls, Minnesota. https://www.replenishliving.com/a-short-history-of-yoga-in-india/#:~:text=The%20practice%20of%20Yoga%20was

McCall, T. (2007, August 28). *38 Health Benefits of Yoga | Yoga Benefits*. Yoga Journal. https://www.yogajournal.com/lifestyle/health/womens-health/count-yoga-38-ways-yoga-keeps-fit/

Michael, (2019, September 19). *The Pineal and Pituitary Glands. Third Eye*. https://temp-empoweryourlifestyles.siterubix.com/pineal-pituitary-glands-purpose-functions-third-eye/

Sovik, R. (2015, May 22). *A Beginner's Guide to Bandhas*. Yogainternational.com; Yoga International. https://yogainternational.com/article/view/a-beginners-guide-to-bandhas

The Real Meaning of Anjali Mudra or "Prayer" Posture. (2020, May 27). Bodhi Surf + Yoga. https://www.bodhisurfyoga.com/meaning-of-anjali-mudra#:~:text=What%20does%20Anjali%20Mudra%20mean

Thomsen, S. (n.d.). *May The Longtime Sun by Sara Thomsen*. Sarathomsen.com. Retrieved May 2, 2021, from https://sarathomsen.com/track/1917667/may-the-longtime-sun

Tomlinson, K. (2017, July 1). *Sun Salutation B sequence with breath*. Ekhart Yoga. https://www.ekhartyoga.com/articles/practice/sun-salutation-b-sequence-with-breath

Wortman, P. (2017, December 6). *The four main bandhas*. Ekhart Yoga. https://www.ekhartyoga.com/articles/practice/the-four-main-bandhas

Yoga Mudra and All Its Benefits: 8 Basic Mudras - BookYogaTeacherTraining.com. (2019). *Yoga Mudra and All Its Benefits: 8 Basic Mudras - BookYogaTeacherTraining.com*. BookYogaTeacherTraining.com. https://www.bookyogateachertraining.com/news/yoga-mudra-and-all-its-benefits

To join June Browne's mailing list, and receive a bonus yoga series for hands and feet, please click or copy this link: https://view.flodesk.com/pages/61fae14 36114df05454c4ed7

Check out June Browne's Author Central page here: https://www.amazon.com/June-Browne/e/B09FGYJ8VT?ref_=dbs_p_e bk_r00_abau_000000

Namaste!

Made in United States
Troutdale, OR
06/09/2023

10517093R00110